Dear Minnie

ALSO BY STACEY DOOLEY

On the Front Line with the Women Who Fight Back
Are You Really OK?: Understanding Britain's Mental Health Emergency

Dear Minnie

Conversations with Remarkable Mothers

Stacey Dooley

BBC Books

UK | USA | Canada | Ireland | Australia
India | New Zealand | South Africa

BBC Books is part of the Penguin Random House group of companies
whose addresses can be found at global.penguinrandomhouse.com

Penguin Random House UK
One Embassy Gardens, 8 Viaduct Gardens, London SW11 7BW

penguin.co.uk
global.penguinrandomhouse.com

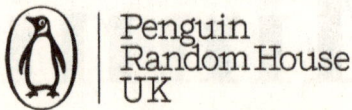
Penguin
Random House
UK

First published by BBC Books in 2025

3

Copyright © Stacey Dooley 2025

First published by BBC Books in 2025

www.penguin.co.uk

A CIP catalogue record for this book is available from the British Library

ISBN 9781785948930

Typeset in 11.5/18.4pt Garamond MT Std by Jouve (UK), Milton Keynes

Printed and bound in Great Britain by Clays Ltd, Elcograf S.p.A.

The authorised representative in the EEA is Penguin Random House Ireland,
Morrison Chambers, 32 Nassau Street, Dublin D02 YH68

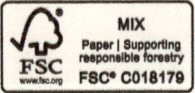
MIX
Paper | Supporting
responsible forestry
FSC® C018179

Penguin Random House is committed to a sustainable future
for our business, our readers and our planet. This book is made
from Forest Stewardship Council® certified paper.

To King Kev and Minnie, our little werewolf
('I'm NOT a good girl, I'm a werewolf').
What a little gang we've made!

Contents

Introduction *1*

Part I: Pregnancy

1. 'If you tell me I can't do something,
I will find a way.'
A story of overcoming the odds 13

2. 'It was all over. I finally had my baby.'
A story of resilience 25

3. 'It was like moving to another country
and knowing you could never move back.'
A story of unexpected fortune 37

4. 'I am part of a club no one wants to belong to.'
A story of loss 51

5. 'It felt like especially precious cargo.'
A story of surrogacy 59

6. 'Who gets the opportunity to go
on maternity leave together?'
A story of shared motherhood 67

Part II: Birth

7. 'You were and will always be the
best surprise we'll ever have.'
A story of teenage motherhood 79

8. 'I knew I was one of the lucky ones.'
A story of courage 89

9. 'I am the mum you deserve to have.'
A story of growth 97

10. 'So off I went to throw my best moves
on the dance floor.'
A story of unexpected labour 105

11. 'Watching you grow is the
most wonderful gift.'
A story of discovery 113

12. 'No matter the journey,
we are perfect for each other.'
A story of adoption 123

Part III: Parenthood

13. 'You showed me that my body
can give me the greatest gift of all.'
A story of recovery 135

14. 'I have never seen you properly,
and I will never see you properly,
but I know every inch of you.'
A story of tenacity 143

15. 'Some days, I feel like we are battling
against the tide.'
A story of strength 153

16. 'I try to remind myself these days are short.'
A story of sleep deprivation 161

17. 'I hope you both have a stable life.'
A story of hope 169

18. 'My purpose was to be a constant presence.'
A story of friendship 175

19. 'I started to imagine myself
as a knight about to ride into battle.'
A story of a working mum 181

20. 'I didn't think this kind of happiness existed.'
A story of reflection 191

Afterword *201*

Resources *203*

Acknowledgements *213*

Introduction

Dear Minnie,

My darling baby girl.

It's 9.10pm, and you are STILL in the bath downstairs with Nanny. Your teeth have been giving you hassle all day, and you've had the hump. But we have had a nap since then, and you are back on form. For now.

I'm upstairs in the office, and your dad is down in London presenting an award at the Palladium. Fancy. Wearing six-inch high heels. (He's playing a drag queen next month and is desperate to nail his walk . . .) He turned the house upside down earlier, trying to find them. 'WHO'S MOVED MY HEELS?!' Spoiler: they were in his wardrobe. How unexpected. :)

My sweetheart Minnie, it's tricky to know where to even begin with this letter. How do I go about trying to tell you what you mean to me? I well up every time I try even to describe the love I hold for you. My little showstopper. My best, best little pal. The love of my life.

Let me fill you in and talk you through when I found out I was preggers. I sort of knew, to be honest. Even before I took the test. I did. I just knew. I just had this instinctive feeling.

I'd been working in town and had finished early enough to go and have a nose around Selfridges. I went and had noodles in the food hall, and then I was just mooching around and completely coincidentally ended up near the chemist concession.

I remember buying the pink toothpaste that I'm into and then going up to the pharmacist, standing behind the till, and very quietly asking for a pregnancy test. I don't remember feeling particularly nervous, but I must've been trying to appear discreet. The lady was such a goodie; she obvs realised I was trying to buy it low-key and offered to staple shut the top of the paper bag, so no one could see what was in it. How thoughtful; I owe her a massive thank you the next time I'm there. I went downstairs for a wee and completely calmly took the test in a Selfridges cubicle. The toilets were heaving: people in every toilet, and a big queue waiting, too.

POSITIVE.

I knew it!

And looking back, sitting here now, it's bonkers, really. What kind of idiot walks into perhaps one of the most recognisable stores in the world and takes the test there if they want to keep it quiet for a while? Me, clearly. I remember calmly pulling my jeans up and exhaling. And feeling quietly delighted and a bit wired! And hot. It's so bloody hot in those loos. Some of my pals tell me of their sheer disbelief when finding out. I didn't really feel that. Like I said, it was more like confirmation.

FAAAAAAAACK, a baby?!!

How exciting! And how MASSIVE! (A deal, not me . . . at this point anyway . . .)

Your dad was filming a series for ITV at the time. I jumped in a black cab and texted him. I can't remember exactly whether I typed 'I'm pregnant' or whether I sent a photo of the test itself, but I vaguely recall him thinking I was taking the piss. And then him realising, 'Wait, are you for real? Like, are you being serious???!'

Dear Minnie

I think he FaceTimed me straight away, but we couldn't really talk too freely because he had a radio mic on, since he was filming this gig. So, it was just the pair of us, staring at each other and, like, whispering and mouthing, 'Are you OK?!' 'Do you feel OK?!' and 'What the fuck?!' to one another. And that was when I started to feel super emotional.

I couldn't have picked a better man to be your dad, honestly.

But the whole moment was so chaotic and grabbed. Simultaneously, the cabby was really kicking off with another cabby, like, super animated, winding the window down and telling him to learn how to fuckin' drive, blah blah blahhhh. Almost squaring up to this other guy.

He was already pissed off; we were living in south-east London, and he didn't wanna go south of the river, so it was hilariously quite the saga. Your dad was like, 'Where are you? What's going on?'

I watch pregnancy reveals on Insta of glossy girls gently calling their boyfriends into their perfectly curated, silent room to hand-deliver the test. None of that perfection with us, I'm afraid.

So that night, your dad was on the telly and it was live, and when the camera passed him, he looked straight down the lens and mouthed, 'I love you Stace,' and I thought, 'NO ONE KNOWS I'M PREGNANT, this is the coolest most special little secret!'

We didn't tell anyone for months except our immediate family and my pal Harriet, whom I trust entirely. I went for dinner with her, and I just really couldn't keep it in. She cried happy tears. And then, very quickly, she turned her attention to the hot young waiter. Good for you, babe.

With our parents, your grandparents, I was in the States working and your dad was up north. So we were trying to make the timings work to FaceTime them because I was eight hours behind. We eventually arranged a time, and I was in a hotel room in Memphis when we told Grandma and Grandad, and Nanny and Grandad. They were ELATED. Couldn't believe it. I had a travel day the following day, and went out that night with my crew and danced all night long in the streets to celebrate. Everyone was drunk, and I was showing off dancing, with my can of sparkling water.

But with everybody else, we were super low-key. On reflection, I wonder if we didn't want to get our hopes up and get too carried away. I was super mindful that miscarriage was a very real possibility. And I certainly didn't want the tabloid press to find out early-ish doors, and then, God forbid, something happened, and we would've been forced into trying to navigate our way through that. And also, it was our news to deliver when we wanted to.

As the months passed, my morning sickness worsened and my boobs were so bloody enormous. We decided it was time to let the cat out the bag (and assure everyone I hadn't had my tits done in LA). Everyone was delighted! Even complete strangers were so bloody kind. The internet really can be the pits sometimes, but the news you were coming brought the good out of all of those lovely people we didn't even know. They were thrilled for us.

As your due date loomed, your daddy and I had done very little, in all honesty, to get ourselves prepared! I was filming with Ukrainian civilians being trained by the British army (waddling around a freezing cold field, dodging grenades, eight months preggers) and your dad was preparing to go on tour, playing a role he'd always dreamt of playing.

It's hardly the generic run-up, but that's how it played out!

Dear Minnie

We couldn't WAIT to meet you and see your stunning little face. (We knew you were beautiful from your 4D scan . . .)

Christmas passed, and 10 January came. The day that changed my life immeasurably.

The day I became your mum. What I've done to deserve you, I'll never know. A love was unlocked that I didn't recognise. It's such an obvious declaration of love, but fuck, it's true, baby! YOU KNOCKED ME OFF MY FEET!

I will love you until the day I die and beyond.

But for now, do me a favour, sweetheart, and get to bed! I'm knackered!

Mummy x

***

THE MOMENT I MET MY Minnie, my life changed immeasurably. I'm SO aware that this sounds so over-the-top dramatic (and painfully predictable!) but honest to God, I really did become a different woman. Maybe (hopefully) a slightly better version of myself? I don't know. I'm deeply grateful to Minnie for that, among many other things. The obvious declarations of love are true, of course, but what I hadn't anticipated was how she would make me feel about other people too. Motherhood has meant I look at almost everyone through a different lens now. It's made me properly see the world and everyone in it. I have this noticeable affection and love for others, even strangers. So unexpected. Now, whenever I look at someone, I see them as somebody else's Minnie. I know this probably sounds a bit mad and a bit right-on, but it's the truth. I have spent so many years throughout my career, hanging out with so many different mums from all over the world, often in extraordinary circumstances. Now I'm a mum myself; it's true I have a newfound, deeper understanding of how being a mum changes almost everything and everyone. And I have an even deeper appreciation for those women. Truly.

I was apprehensive when putting pen to paper, as I really didn't want to focus only on my own experiences and point of view. Obviously, I am DEFINITELY NO EXPERT, so I for sure didn't want to present myself as someone with (any) all of the answers! God, I wish I had them! I never read one pregnancy or baby book (despite my very thoughtful neighbour lending me all the literature she swore by). I didn't listen to any podcasts and didn't visit a single NCT class. To say I went in clueless would be the understatement of the year. I know lots of people swear by all the preparations, but for me, it just really wouldn't have been my scene, I don't think. We ended up just winging it, which was both hilarious and ridiculous. So, when it came to this book, it was important to me to explore motherhood through the eyes of many different mums. And I can't tell you how grateful I am that they were so bloody generous and forthcoming. Thank you.

I am very mindful that motherhood is different for every person who experiences it. I am also acutely aware that my pregnancy and birth were relatively straightforward. I have help emotionally, and financially I am secure. I am supported and looked after by my partner, our families and our pals. I know that is not how it always plays out, so I thought I would try to get an insight into what motherhood looks and feels like for different mums. I am delighted that we managed to connect with and speak to many amazing women from all walks of life who have had many different experiences, including an incredibly impressive mum who is blind and works as a barrister, a mum who fled the Democratic Republic of the Congo who opened up so candidly about the stark differences between her own childhood and that of her kids, and a mum who turned her life around so she could finally be the mother she wanted to be to her kids.

I decided to divide the book into three sections – pregnancy, birth and parenthood. Motherhood is an extraordinary journey (I mean, I hate the 'J' word but in this case it's so bloody true) that starts long before the incredible sound of a newborn's cries fills the delivery room. For some, like Hannah, a midwife we spoke to, it is a path of endurance, marked by the challenges of fertility treatments, and the emotional highs and lows of hoping, waiting and praying for a baby. And some, like the lovely Stacey, who went through early menopause, are determined to become a mother, however it happens.

Often when women are pregnant, there is such a focus on the birth. Frequently, I think the birth plan goes out the window almost the minute you are in the delivery room – so I was keen to have a story of a birth that did not go to plan, and Lizzie came up trumps with her story about her waters breaking on a party boat. But of course, motherhood encompasses more than just birth; it includes the countless moments that follow. I was also determined to include stories of adoption and surrogacy, and debunk the myth of stepmotherhood, a role which is often reduced to lazy generalisations.

I loved the idea of love letters from mums to their kids. Featuring letters to start chapters of the book felt like a fantastic way of giving these mothers a voice and complete control over what they wanted to say to their children. It also opened people up to speak to me about their experiences with such honesty. Letters are so beautifully personal. I think many of us may not write letters like this anymore (I mean, realistically, when have we got the luxury of time between googling rashes and panicking about the shade of today's shit!), but it is such a special way of articulating emotions and capturing a moment in time. Now my Minnie is a toddler, and it feels like I was pregnant literally a second ago, and I KNOW we are always bombarded with clichés but it's honestly so true when they say you blink and they've grown up. What an incredible gift for these kids in many years to know how their mum felt at that very moment.

It would be impossible to capture every experience; no two mothers are the same. Within the letters – and my conversations with each contributor – there might be sentiments or experiences that you can really connect with and that feel very familiar.

Chatting to these women, there were so many moments when I thought, 'GOD, I so hear you!'

Lauren, who spoke about sleep deprivation with her third child, was one I genuinely could understand. When you're in the trenches of sleep deprivation, you legitimately wonder if you'll ever sleep or feel like you're back in the room again! The first six months, my living room looked like a teenager's bedroom. Cuppas, chocolate and Netflix on a loop, trying to get through those 4am feeds. Other mums have had very unique experiences, and it felt like a real privilege to hear from them, too.

Dear Minnie

At its core, motherhood is about love, right? A profound, indescribable love that knocks you sideways. It sustains us through those bloody hellish sleepless nights, bugs (I wasn't prepared for the constant fevers and infections!), and all the other unexpected challenges, and constantly reminds us how lucky we are to get a shot at this gig. I hope you enjoy this small glimpse into what motherhood can look like.

Part I
Pregnancy

1

'If you tell me I can't do something, I will find a way.'

A story of overcoming the odds

To Sofia,

When I was 29, I was told by the doctor that I was going through the menopause and I wouldn't be able to have children. At first, I was completely numb. I didn't believe what they were saying. Menopause is something older women go through. But then it all made sense. The changes to my body, the overly emotional state I would get into for no reason. The sweating for no reason. For a moment, I forgot about the not being able to have children and felt that it all made sense and I wasn't going mad. Then, it felt like an elephant was sitting on my chest. I couldn't have children. I had always wanted to be a mum, but from then, the want became a need. It consumed me like nothing I could ever put into words. It was all I could think about; I knew what you would look like, how I wanted your nursery to look. I even knew your name. I just knew I needed you; the only thing I didn't know was how this would happen.

For two years, I researched and went to seminars on adoption, fostering, egg and sperm donation, and embryo donation. Even though it would have been an easier option financially and physically to go with an embryo donation, I chose the route of egg and sperm donation. I didn't want someone giving you something that I couldn't – a mum, a dad and siblings – a ready-made family that shares your DNA. I told friends and family what I wanted to do, but when speaking to Grandma's brother, Uncle David, he made me realise that I wasn't alone, and it became a 'how are WE going to make a baby' plan. Between me, Grandma, Uncle David and Aunty Nicky, we set the plan in motion.

During this time, I was working as a live-in nanny. I was very open and honest with the family about my plans and told them that once my contract was up in a few months' time, I wouldn't be going back. It worked well for them, too, as by then, all three of their children were at school full-time. This allowed me to make my hospital appointments around school hours. Once I finished my contract with them, I was introduced to a family with a young baby who were looking for a four-day-week live-out nanny. I told them about my situation, and they were happy for me to pick my day off to fit around hospital appointments.

The doctor told me that I could either use a sperm bank from the UK or one from the USA. I chose the American one, as there was more variety and because it was less likely that you would bump into a sibling. Growing up with my brother, I know the connection we have is a sibling love; I didn't want you to meet a sibling, not know who they were and confuse the connection that you might feel with a romantic love. I went onto the website, and after putting on filters of attributes that I wanted the sperm donor to possess, I got to look through their profiles. It didn't take me too long to pick your donor. He had kind eyes and a warm smile. I then got to go through his medical history, and was able to read a statement he had written about himself. He came across as smart, musical, and someone who loved science and animals. Once you buy the sperm, they release more pictures of your donor from a young age up to the present day. When you give birth, they give you a choice to contact the other mums that used his sperm. I agreed to and am in touch with these women. We share pictures and stories about all of our children, your 'diblings', and if and when you are ready, I will support you in meeting them. You all have the same nose, chin and dimple. I also made sure that I chose a man who would be open to meeting you when you are older. When you are 18, if you want to meet him, I have put money aside to pay for you to go to America. If you decide not to, that money is yours for any adventure you choose.

You don't get to pick the egg donor. I just knew that she needed IVF. We were able to help each other in different ways. She helped me medically, and in return, I helped her financially. All I know about her is that she must have the biggest heart in the world as she helped create you. Just like the man in America, when you are 18, if you choose to meet her, I will be by your side and have as much or as little involvement as you want.

The sperm was flown here and was fertilised with the egg to form an embryo – you in a little dish. I was on lots of medication, and when the lining of my uterus was thick enough, they put you in my tummy. You were the third attempt. I'm so happy that the other times didn't work. Otherwise, I wouldn't have you.

I found out I was pregnant with you in a toilet in a gym. I carried on my morning for about an hour before I told anyone. I just felt calm and at peace. But then it hit me. I was shaking and crying with excitement when I called Grandma. I waited until the next morning before I told everyone else. I took a picture of the pregnancy test and just sent it to everyone who had supported us and our journey so far. They say you should wait until 12 weeks before you tell people, but I needed to say it out loud for it to be real.

Every morning, Grandma would ask me how I felt. I told her sick, and she replied, 'Good. Means it's cooking.' I couldn't wait to find out if you were a boy or a girl, so I had a special scan. At first, they thought you were a boy. I knew they were wrong. They told me to go for a walk, and then they would try again. Yep, I was right; you are a girl. When I FaceTimed Grandma to tell her, she laughed and said, 'You have your best friend for life, but gosh, I hope she brings karma with her.'

Your personality and strong will were evident before you were even born. You never faced the right way for a picture and would only move when you wanted to – and that wasn't that often. So much so that the doctors decided you should be born four weeks early. When you arrived, I couldn't hold you straight away as you needed some help with your breathing. But as soon as I heard you cry, I turned to Grandma and said, 'Now I am complete.'

Now you are five, and your personality is infectious. You love clothes and fashion, and you are always trying to make people laugh, and have empathy like no one else I know. You love movies, especially with ice cream and popcorn. Even though you can play for hours on your own, being surrounded by other children is something you love more than anything, especially in a park.

I once saw a medium who told me that I would meet the love of my life, and they were from across the sea. They were right – part of you comes from across the sea, and you are the love of my life. No one can tell me that because we do not share DNA you are not my child. From the moment you were born, I grew an extra heart, but it was outside of my chest. I don't get people saying we look alike, but as soon as you open your mouth, people always say they know whose kid you are. We really are like two peas in a pod.

Dear Minnie

You are my world, my beating heart, my biggest accomplishment, the best adventure, and my daughter. I love you always.

Love Mum x

***

W HEN I MET STACEY, SHE talked about how she always wanted to be a mum and was very maternal. It did not occur to her before the diagnosis of early menopause that it would not happen for her.

'My mum went through the menopause early, so I should've thought about having tests for it earlier, but I just didn't think,' she said. 'I started having irregular periods and mood swings from when I was about 19, but I put that down to teenage hormones!'

At the time, Stacey was working as a nursery nurse and said that her biggest fear was her fertility.

'I knew I wanted to be a mum myself. I had always said that if I hadn't met anyone by the time I was 36, I would do it on my own. So, the possibility of being a single mum was always at the back of my mind.'

After it was confirmed by her doctor that she had gone through early menopause, and she knew she would struggle to conceive, she felt spurred into action. I could tell just by talking to her what a powerful and single-minded woman she is.

'I am the sort of person who, if you tell me I can't do something, will find a way. So, I did. In the end, I had Sofia at 35, so it wasn't far off what I had planned anyway. Though, of course, the diagnosis affected

17

my dating life before then. At what point do you tell people that you can't have kids? It's hard.'

In 2023, research showed that since 2009, the number of donor-conceived children born in the UK had more than tripled, representing 1 in 170 of all births. According to the Human Fertilisation and Embryology Authority (HFEA), this equates to a couple of donor-conceived children in every primary school. While nearly half of all donor gametes (sperm, eggs, or both) are used by heterosexual couples experiencing male- or female-factor infertility, much of the recent increase, especially in the use of donor sperm, has been driven by women in same-sex relationships and solo mothers.

The growth of new pathways to parenthood is an incredible development. However, as the practice of donor conception – using donor sperm, eggs, or embryos to create a family – becomes more widespread, the associated ethical dilemmas are also growing increasingly complex.

I followed a similar situation to Stacey's a few years ago for my TV show *DNA: Family Secrets*. Arguably, there is more of a focus on sperm donors rather than egg donors. I wonder whether this is because sperm donation is more common than egg donation, and because the demand for sperm donation is generally higher. Sperm donation also has minimal medical risks to the donor, while egg donation is a more invasive procedure.

'I became quite fixated on the whole process, so I did a lot of research,' Stacey told me. 'It's all I could think about. I spoke to doctors and went to seminars. There were so many ways of having a baby with egg and sperm donors, including egg donation, sperm donation, or even embryo adoption, where IVF has been done, and you can "adopt" an embryo.'

Stacey talked through options for egg and sperm donation in the UK and abroad, which also can include anonymous donations. She decided she did not want anonymous donors, so she went onto a list for an egg donor.

In 2005, the UK government amended the law to allow donor-conceived children the legal right to access identifying information about their egg or sperm donors once they turn 18. This legal change has since deterred some potential donors from participating in the donation process, and so there is now a shortage of egg donors in the UK to help infertile women or couples. Many now go abroad to find donor eggs, but Stacey decided to stick to a UK egg donor.

'Most important to me was the egg donor's health. I also wanted a donor with an "open door" so Sofia could look into her ancestry if she ever wanted to. When you look for an egg donor, you go on a list, and you can pick features that you might want. You can give them all the attributes you want the donor to have, such as their eye colour, height, and so on. Obviously, the more things you require, the longer it will take to get a donor match. That means as soon as you get to the top of the list and the donor doesn't match your criteria, you get moved down. They told me it could be anywhere between 6 months and 18 months. I have red hair and brown eyes, and I could've said I wanted a donor with the same features. There is also the religious factor; I am Jewish, so ideally, I would've loved a Jewish donor, but that would've put me back years. I was so eager that I didn't put much on my list, and I found a profile that matched what I was looking for in nine months.'

Stacey said that her only fear is that when and if her daughter goes looking for her biological mum, she might not be interested in getting to know her.

'I am not scared of them opening their arms to her because it is another person to love her, and I am still her mum. It was my choice to have her in this way – it will then be her choice. I will always support and respect her decisions.'

Stacey chose a US sperm donor, so there is less chance of her daughter 'bumping into a sibling without realising'. At the last count, Sofia has 16 'diblings', mainly living in America, Canada and Australia. She says the majority of the families talk to each other and exchange information about their children. There is only one other family that used the same donor in the UK, who Stacey met up with a few weeks before we spoke.

'Before we met, I was fascinated to see how the kids would interact with each other and by the science of it all,' she explained in a matter-of-fact tone. 'Sofia can be quite shy at first when she meets new people, and then her personality comes out, so I was interested to see how quickly she would feel at ease with the other child.

'I was quite nervous and thought about cancelling it, but I plucked up the courage. They had the same nose, dimple and chin – all 16 of them have that feature. Personality-wise, they were polar opposites. That's why I wanted to go and see whether it is nature or nurture. In this case, it is definitely nurture!'

Stacey said that people tell her Sofia looks like her 'all the time'.

'I don't think she necessarily looks like me, but she has my mannerisms,' Stacey explained. 'She says things, and with her mannerisms like the way she laughs; it just looks like me! She is just beyond!'

Even if we are not affected by infertility, most of us will know someone who is. The World Health Organization (WHO) says that one in six people globally is affected by infertility. The WHO recommends that countries provide universal health coverage for fertility treatments, following the model set by Denmark, Sweden, Indonesia, Spain and Morocco, which support their citizens through their healthcare systems. Accessing fertility treatment can be challenging for people who do not live in these countries. In the UK, NHS-funded IVF cycles are available to some people. However, access is limited due to various factors, including restrictions, and it often comes down to a postcode lottery. According to recent data from the Human Fertilisation and Embryology Authority, the number of NHS-funded IVF cycles has been declining across the UK since 2019.

The process of IVF cost Stacey £23,000, but of course, Sofia is 'utterly priceless'.

'It's a lot of money. The lottery for IVF is that you have to fit into so many boxes,' Stacey explained. 'Because I am single, I wouldn't have been able to get IVF anyway, and because it is an egg donor, they don't do that on the NHS. I was never going to be able to do anything through the NHS.'

Stacey had help from family members and saved up as much as she could. 'The costs added up because things went wrong. My daughter was conceived during my third round.'

We talked about how opinions have changed towards single mums and donor conceptions.

'I used to have people ask, "What happened?" or "Where's her dad?" I was pretty straight with them and told them that I chose to be a single mum. When they told me I was brave, I felt it was quite patronising.

'Now it is a lot more common. My uncle just called me this morning, asking if I can chat with one of his work colleagues who is thinking about trying to have a baby on her own.'

When Sofia was about three or four, they were in the car together and she asked Stacey if 'she grew in her tummy and how she got there'.

'Her tone was very matter-of-fact. I'm sure my heart stopped for a second or two.'

Stacey told Sofia about how she was conceived and plans to tell her daughter more about the situation as she gets older.

'I told her that Mummy wasn't able to have children, so a really nice man, an amazing woman and a great doctor came together to help her have her. That's the story we go with now, and she doesn't ask any questions.'

Even though Stacey is described on paper as a 'single mum', she says she does not feel like this. In the way she spoke about the people who have supported her, I could feel the warmth and closeness of her family.

'My mum let me move back home with her when I was pregnant. She is very much a part of my daughter's life, as are my aunts, uncles, cousins and brother. If I ask Sofia if she wants a dad or siblings, she will always say no. When I ask her why, she tells me: "I've got a mum and a grandma – that's enough." She's very happy, and I want to support her in the way my family has supported me.'

I have a bit of a soft spot for single mums. I was raised by my mum for the first few years of my life. Doing those first few days/weeks/months alone must've been relentless. My nan was very hands-on, though. She was the landlady of a pub miles away from Luton, so of course we weren't seeing her every day, but she would send parcels and come and stay and help out whenever she could. And we'd go up to her pub a lot. I actually have beautiful, very clear memories of hanging out with her. She was FUN. Her name was Hazel, and everyone called her

'Crazy Haze'. She was in love with Tina Turner and the host of legendary lock-ins. It was my job to straighten the Orangina bottles and clean the ashtrays. Light work! It was clear to me, chatting with Stacey, how strong the female bonds in her family are.

It's funny how history repeats itself as I watch my daughter with my mum. Minnie is obsessed with her Nanny, and my mum is equally smitten with her. She is incredibly hands-on and helps a lot, especially when I'm working. She spoils Minnie rotten with treats, but also time. She's so playful with her and I do feel so lucky that they have that relationship.

It's ironic, you spend your formative years not wanting to be anywhere near your mum, and then you have a baby, and they are the only other person you truly trust with your child! Hilarious really.

Obviously, it's not genetics alone that make you a mum. Sometimes I look at Minnie and she's my double, but there are other occasions she's all Kev. In terms of her character, she's me all over. Every morning, she literally prises my lids open: 'Mummy, get up now, good morning, put your clothes on!' And from that moment on, I am being bossed around. She's mischievous and funny. She's always trying to negotiate with me. My hustler.

I am so mindful that I have my boyfriend, my mum and Kev's mum to help look after Minnie. It's definitely a team effort, and the whole family is so hands-on and really involved in raising Minnie. But for all mums, we all know that there are some days when you can feel like you are going to run out of steam. The proverb that it 'takes a village to raise a child' is definitely true. In countries such as China and Vietnam, co-parenting with grandparents is common. Recent studies in several Asian nations have shown that the support, role modelling, and encouragement provided by extended family can help new mothers feel more confident in their parenting roles. While Western parents may approach parenting differently, this does not necessarily make their methods right or wrong. But I do believe that bringing up a family has to be easier if you have family and friends who are around you and can help.

It also helps with the cost of childcare, which can be prohibitive for so many mothers in the UK who want to work but can't afford to. Under a law passed in Sweden in December 2023, parents are now allowed to allocate a portion of their parental leave to grandparents during their child's first year, so essentially, they are paid to care for their grandkids. It's interesting that Sweden was the first country to introduce paid parental leave for fathers in 1974 and many countries have followed; I hope the same happens in this case.

It was clear Stacey has all the support she needs – and that Sofia is growing up into a gorgeous little girl.

'Oh, don't get me wrong,' Stacey said, laughing with a low cackle. 'I do get time for myself. I am going away in a few weeks with just my girl-friends. All mums need a break. We have days now where she is happy to play by herself, and more than that, she's become a friend now. We go out shopping together, and she tells me what goes with what and if it looks nice, like my very own personal shopper. Every Saturday night, we have a movie night together with pizza on the sofa; she picks the movie, and we have some microwave popcorn. She has my sense of humour and gets sarcasm. We laugh non-stop. It's like having a pal.'

2

'It was all over.
I finally had my baby.'

A story of resilience

Dear Kasper,

I wonder if, by the time you read this, you will know how desperately wanted you were? Will you know how much we hoped, how long we waited and how hard we tried for you? Will you know how Daddy kept my heart from breaking when I thought it would crumble to dust?

When we decided to try for a baby, I was 30 and working as a midwife. We didn't meet you for another five years, after countless attempts and failures at IVF. I was so panicked that I might never have a baby; it was absolutely all-consuming, even though I tried to be grateful for our lovely life. Trying for a baby became who I was and what I did. There wasn't a minute it wasn't on my mind. If I wasn't talking about it, I was thinking about it. I was going to work every day. The cruel irony slapped me in the face on every shift I worked! A woman who helps bring babies into the world couldn't make or carry one herself.

I worked on the birth centre and was delivering babies all the time. I used to find it very emotional to see a family being created right in front of me. I used to feel envious of the love and happiness. But I can honestly say I never felt cheated that people were having babies, and I wasn't. They weren't my family; it wasn't my baby; people's circumstances are so different. So, there wasn't a time when I thought I would swap everything we had for a baby because I knew that Daddy and I would be happy, and at that time, that's all I had to hold on to. All this being said, the feelings of failure were real and chipped away at my self-esteem. These feelings have always stayed with me, and I am always wondering if I am good enough for you. But perhaps this is the thought of mothers the world over?

I didn't find the physical side of IVF treatment very difficult. The process became a job to do, a task to complete, a hurdle to overcome. Everything else we did was an attempt to distract us from the reality of our situation. What was hard was that I felt from the beginning that I always had to bang on the door, trying to advocate for myself for the investigations I wanted. I was well informed, and we were so lucky to be able to afford treatment, but it seemed to be a 'one-size-fits-all' approach. I'm sure you can imagine how that went down with me! I was persistent in phoning for cancellations so that I might be seen sooner. I took matters into my own hands to have some tests that the doctor said I didn't need, and thank goodness I did. Otherwise, we would have been waiting another few years, I am sure of it.

Daddy always says I was so strong and confident in my approach, but it was because I was desperate. By the time I got pregnant, I was very disconnected from the little embryo that started to grow.

Pregnancy was a means to an end, I'm afraid; I just couldn't relax. Although as the time to your birth came nearer, I'd let myself get a bit excited . . . but I kept that feeling a secret. I thought if I showed it and then you didn't arrive, I'd feel so embarrassed that I'd failed at the final hurdle. Your birth was eventful as I had pre-eclampsia, a planned caesarean and then a few complications with the operation. It was very strange being on the receiving end of care, and I was extremely nervous. I was shaking all over, and my heart was beating so fast. It was completely surreal. When you finally arrived, our ninth little embryo, you felt like a miracle! When they lifted you up, I can remember a wave of utter relief that all the trying was over, I'd done it, and I'd made it . . . I was finally the same as everyone else.

Throughout our fertility treatments and pregnancies, your daddy was so strong. I don't think he ever wavered in his resolve and belief that you'd arrive one day. He was absolutely smitten with you and has been ever since. I couldn't believe he loved you so much so quickly. I remember lying on the theatre table, looking at Daddy's face, and feeling like he'd gone to another planet!

It took me a little while longer to get used to you. In fact, I think it took us a little time to get used to each other. I hadn't dared believe you could be real while you were in my tummy, and so when you came, I wasn't sure who I was, who you were or what we were supposed to do together.

Breastfeeding you was very difficult for about six weeks; you were early, tiny and tongue-tied. I was a bit crazy! My midwife head went foggy, and I found myself in the position that I had been so scared of: what if I couldn't breastfeed you? This was so important to me, and I thought I'd be good at it. I remember thinking that it was another thing I'd failed at. I was so frustrated one night that I put you down and shouted at you. I didn't know how to help you. I was very lucky to have two amazing colleagues who helped me get the hang of it, and I really believe that being able to breastfeed you for a whole year helped to heal some of the hurt and feelings of failure.

My darling, we figured it out, and I have grown with you. Waiting for you taught me patience and an ability to accept sadness. It taught me to look outward, beyond myself. I have been learning from you for such a long time, Kasper.

As I write this, you are two years old. Gorgeous, funny and stubborn. I love you more and more as you grow. I don't know how other mothers feel, but for me, my love over-flows for you and seems to expand with time as you become a little person. How much will I love you when you are a grown man if this continues?! Maybe that's nature's way of helping mothers cope with the passing of time.

I hope my love shines out of you and polishes you with joy and kindness as you go through your life. Most of all, I hope that you are happy, my baby.

With all my love.

I am forever yours,

Mama

***

I WONDER WHETHER LOTS OF women like me feel that it is at the age of 35 that we might start running into complications when it comes to getting pregnant? We are all told that our fertility falls off a cliff then, and our most fertile years are over. But it's more nuanced than that – a woman's peak fertility years are typically from her late teens to late twenties. Around age 30, fertility begins to gradually decline, with the rate of decline accelerating in the mid-thirties. However, the reduc-tion in the likelihood of pregnancy after age 35 is more of a gradual slope than a sudden drop, continuing in this gradual way until around age 40.

Female babies are born with all the eggs they will ever have – approximately 2 million – but by puberty, this number has already dropped to about 600,000. The ovarian reserve continues to diminish throughout adulthood. As women age, both the quantity and quality of their eggs decline, making natural conception more challenging. This decrease in egg quality and quantity means that even with fertility treatments, the overall success rates may be lower compared to when a woman is younger. It is widely understood that the decline in egg quality and quantity accelerates after age 35, but the rate of decline can vary from person to person.

Many of my pals have had IVF, and they all have had babies. I can see from their experiences that it's definitely complex. I assumed that I would probably need IVF, because I started trying for a baby quite late, but I was lucky to fall pregnant with Minnie quickly. We don't know if it will be so easy the second time, and it might still be something we will need to do in the future.

Since 1991, over 1.3 million IVF cycles and more than 260,000 donor insemination (DI) cycles have been performed in the UK, resulting in the birth of 390,000 babies, according to new figures from the Human Fertilisation and Embryology Authority (HFEA). The fertility regulator's annual Fertility Trends report, published in the organisation's thirtieth anniversary year, highlights the advances and changes in fertility treatment over the past three decades. The report shows that IVF cycles have increased significantly, from 6,700 in 1991 to over 69,000 in 2019. This is due to a combination of factors, including rapid growth in development and innovation across the sector, making the process safer and more effective. There is now greater awareness of IVF and fertility treatments, which has helped reduce stigma and encouraged more people to seek help, and many people are choosing to have children later in life, which can have an impact on fertility. There are also many more centres and clinics, making it much more accessible.

I wanted to include a story of someone who had IVF after struggling to conceive. Hannah's perspective as a midwife added a new dimension to her struggle, as she constantly interacted with newborn babies and mothers.

'For me now, it's just what happened to me. Looking back, I realise what a hard time it was,' she said quietly. 'I was always trying to downplay it and make it OK for everyone else, especially my family. I really wanted to protect them all the time. My mum and sister, particularly, I couldn't bear the thought of them seeing how sad I was about it. The only person who saw me at my lowest was my husband. I think my family knew how hard it was for me to manage, and they were very supportive. I talked about it, quite practically, but I never let on how I really felt. I couldn't face putting it on them.'

Hannah told me how she got through IVF by treating it as a prac-tical task like her work – with her husband 'dragging her along (in a good way)'.

I understand a bit of what it entails from speaking with friends: injecting yourself with several types of medication, enduring endless prodding as the sonographer determines if your lining is perfect and your follicles are the ideal size. Then, it's time to go under anaesthesia while your eggs are collected. The eggs are fertilised in the lab and you'll spend the next few days anxiously jumping every time the phone rings as you wait to hear which embryos made the cut, until the time comes to put them back in again. And then after that, the two-week wait to see if it was successful.

From talking to people undergoing IVF treatment, it seems that it can feel like everyone around them is getting pregnant easily and giving birth. In addition to helping mums give birth to babies every day at work, Hannah's two sisters-in-law had two children, each within 18 months, so it was very hard for her to escape the excitement of new babies in her home and working lives: 'There were four new grandchildren in the family in less time than I had been trying for one baby.'

Hannah's story reminded me of a documentary I watched, *Alex Jones: Making Babies*, in which Jones interviewed a paediatrician struggling to get pregnant. This doctor spent her life helping other people's kids, and like Hannah, who was spending her days delivering other people's children, this seemed like a particularly cruel twist of fate.

'I really liked my job but by the time I went on maternity leave, I couldn't wait to get out of there. When I went off from work, there were still the relics of Covid-19 regulations, and you could work from home from 28 weeks pregnant while doing administrative work. My husband asked if I would be bored, but I couldn't wait to leave. I was on the birth centre and loved that, but I wouldn't say I liked it by then. It wasn't because I didn't love looking after the ladies; I just couldn't believe that my own pregnancy was real.'

When she fell pregnant, Hannah said, she presumed she would find the experience of early motherhood easy.

'I was fine, really, but it never occurred to me that I would find it difficult or that I would not bond very well with him at first,' she explained candidly. 'It never even entered my head. Now I know I wasn't really connected with him when I was pregnant. I was very standoffish about the whole thing.'

As an insider looking in, having IVF appears to be very taxing emotionally and, at times, it can feel all-consuming. Speaking to my mates who have been through IVF, I know some of them never wanted to allow themselves to get excited or carried away, in case their hopes would come crashing down again.

Hannah added thoughtfully: 'The whole thing was surreal. I had him at work, and when they told me I was going to the theatre to have a spinal, where I go every day for work to do them for other women, I didn't really let myself think it was going to happen. I could not believe a baby would come. When he arrived, the overwhelming feeling was relief that it was over – it was all over. The whole thing. Finally, I had my baby.'

Hannah then talked about her experience of early motherhood and getting to grips with everything that entailed, like breastfeeding, which was really important to her.

'I was hellbent on doing it,' Hannah told me, and I could see the determination in her face. 'I think it was psychological. My sister, sisters-in-law, and most of my friends had done it. They all managed to get pregnant, and nearly all of them managed to have vaginal births. I felt there was a lot tied to breastfeeding for me – I couldn't get pregnant, then I couldn't have a vaginal birth, so I *had* to be able to breastfeed.

'At the beginning, Kasper was really small and jaundiced, and milk was pouring over his face. He couldn't get it in his mouth. I was fortunate – I had two colleagues who helped me. One of them is a very good friend who came on two Sundays in a row and stayed all day to help me. We just kept trying. I was so lucky I had her, because I kept going. In the end, it was really healing for me to be able to do it.'

Hannah took additional time off work after her statutory maternity leave and has really enjoyed returning to midwifery.

'Being back and enjoying my job again has been really lovely. I feel like I have gone back with a bit more ambition to move forward in my career,' she said in an upbeat tone. 'For a long time, I felt like the only way to move forward was to have a baby. I was really stuck.'

Hannah also felt she now has a different view of breastfeeding after finding it tricky.

'Where I work in Bradford is a very diverse population, so doing my job, I'm aware of the different cultures and situations. It's given me a new perspective on breastfeeding and how we can help women with it. I really don't think – from my experience – that there is pressure from midwives to breastfeed. We can't promote formula in any way, but I don't think there is pressure from us for mums to breastfeed because it is the choice of the individual. If the mum wants to breast-feed and it's straightforward, and the mum finds it relatively easy to get started, we can help. But if the mums run into trouble and they are at home, it is difficult for them to get the specialist help they need to breastfeed successfully.

'The women who can afford it will seek it out, but it is often the women who need it most, where there are health inequalities, and they do not have as much money to find someone who could help them – they are the ones who could really benefit from more support.'

The UK has some of the lowest breastfeeding rates globally. UNICEF data reveals that in England, the rate of exclusive breastfeeding falls from 81 per cent at birth to 24 per cent at six weeks and then to 17 per cent at three months. It says that eight out of ten women stop before they want to. I know some women find breastfeeding challenging, and the topic is so emotive. We talked a bit about the issues around feeding your baby, including the fact it can still be frowned upon to breastfeed when you are out and about, even though mothers are protected in public places. I read about one scheme in Derby that helped women overcome feeling uncomfortable or awkward about breastfeeding, with businesses and organisations hanging up signs saying, 'Breastfeeding welcome here.' In turn, it was hoped that this would boost the businesses as breastfeeding mums would feel happy to return because they felt comfortable.

I never thought I would breastfeed – I felt it was a bit woo-woo – but for me, it's been one of the best things I have ever done. As soon as they placed Minnie on my chest, she literally went down to my boob. They wheeled me down the corridor, and I was waving at everyone with my tits out. I was very lucky. In the early days, I did worry about whether she was getting enough milk; I didn't know what I was doing, and it was pretty full-on, but it seemed to work. There was one boob that was always full, and the other wasn't – so I did have wonky tits for a while. Kev thought it was hilarious; it was like they belonged to two different women! Minnie was breastfed for about 14 months. After a year, I wanted to stop; I was knackered, but weaning her off was also a saga. If we have another baby, I'd definitely want to do it again. It's so funny how this time around it would be so important to me. Of course, it's personal, and of course, it's not always possible . . . but for me, I'm made up we went down that road. (Apart from the leaking in public – urgh, what a palaver!)

'My experience has really given me more understanding in my work,' Hannah added. 'And this is so valuable.'

3

'It was like moving to another country and knowing you could never move back.'

A story of unexpected fortune

My darling boys,

I can't start your story without telling you about the babies that came before you, the ones that didn't make it. Saying goodbye to them not only broke my heart but broke my soul. When I said goodbye to my first baby, I wrote her a letter, a bit like this; it was the first time I'd ever signed 'Mummy', and it was a goodbye letter. That day, I felt winded by a mix of such intense grief and love. The extremes of two wild emotions that shouldn't be served up together. I loved her so much, she was part of me, and I wasn't ready to say goodbye. We should have just been starting out together. When I buried her, I screamed like only a mother can.

It was a dark time, physically, mentally and spiritually. But through all that pain, I never stopped believing in you. I knew you were coming. When I was lying in hospital on my own, not allowed any visitors because of Covid-19, coming round after having my second baby surgically removed, I knew with unwavering conviction you were coming to me, and I would keep going.

And around six months later, I was pregnant again.

I was excited but frightened that this pregnancy would end like my last two. This wasn't helped by the fact that at a very early scan I had, they couldn't even see that you were there! They told me it could be an ectopic pregnancy and sent me home with an alarming leaflet.

At the next scan, on Christmas Eve 2021, there you were: a grey swishing blob on the screen, like a creature from the deep. I couldn't tell what I was looking at, but the consultant told me I had two babies.

I still remember looking straight into your dad's eyes and seeing his tears. You know, he's not an emotional man, but that moment was such a special surprise. We had prepared ourselves for bad news, and you know him – he's a professional sceptic – but we got a miracle. The doctors were very cautious and told me there was 'no guarantee' that you'd make it, especially with my history and age (I was 38 at the time).

They gave me drugs to take, and I did everything by the book. You name it – I even stopped drinking coffee, and you know how seriously I take my coffee drinking. I just wanted to do all I could to keep you.

In January, we had a scan to determine heartbeats. We'd never got heartbeats before; this had always been the end of the road. I was holding my breath and praying. Your dad had Covid, so he couldn't come in with me. He had to wait in the car park with Wilbur (our dog).

Petrified but trying not to cry, I went into the scan on my own. I got on the bed and closed my eyes. But I knew something was up; the sonographer called the consultant over. It took DEEP faith not to panic at that moment, just to close my eyes and count my breaths.

The consultant said, 'We have healthy heartbeats,' and I felt like I could finally breathe. Like all the tension and fear that start in that place in your stomach, where you feel sick, released. But there was a 'but'.

She flipped the monitor around, and I again saw a blobby, blurry outline. She pointed to three tiny moving white blobs – pumping hearts. I went into a paralysing shock. I couldn't even get dressed. She kept telling me, 'It's time to put your knickers on now.' It took a long time to sink in, especially for your dad. I got back in the car and said, 'It's good news, but can you drive somewhere we can talk properly?'

He clocked that I had three pieces of paper in my hand – medical reports. Then I said, 'It's good news, but there are three heartbeats.'

His instant reaction was 'Oh no' – I think because of all the very serious risks of complications this came with. We didn't tell anyone else for a while as we needed some time to get our heads around it.

Even through the pregnancy, the whole thing felt so surreal. I remember saying to another parent that it felt like I was about to get a one-way ticket to another country where I didn't speak the language or understand the culture. It was all so alien and permanent. I knew life wouldn't be the same, but I didn't know exactly what it would be like.

The whole way through the pregnancy, we were very aware that things could go wrong. I was high risk. I remember being at a midwife appointment and actually seeing red flags all over my records. It was a very anxious time. I really worked hard to stay calm because I didn't want to flood you with stress hormones. I meditated, used breathing techniques and had the support of a wonderful group of spiritual women.

But there were naysayers — doom-mongers who would remind me of all the horrendous risks I was exposed to, all the horrible things that could happen to you (and me). This started with the doctors but seeped out into the family. I had to hold firm and tell them, 'Right now, I have healthy babies who can hear you doubting them.'

The doctors even suggested I 'terminate' one of you at our 12-week scan. This scan lasted three hours, and I had a panic attack within the first hour. I was so utterly desperate for them to tell me you were OK, and they wouldn't say anything until their boss, the consultant, came in at the end. When she finally turned up, she frightened us with complications and syndromes I'd never heard of.

Then she told us that we could potentially lower the risks of these awful things happening if we terminated one of you. They call this 'selective reduction'. I couldn't believe she was actually suggesting I kill one of my babies. I'd just buried two! I told her there was no way and got very upset. Yet she persisted in discussing statistics with your dad. I was outraged that two people who weren't carrying you were having a conversation about 'terminating' one of you. I felt powerless and angry. There was no F-ing way I was going to let anything happen to you.

I knew there was a lot I needed to organise, but we didn't want to start buying things until we'd reached the end of the second trimester.

Dear Minnie

I don't enjoy shopping and found it completely bamboozling. I didn't know what half the products were or if we really needed them, and then I felt like a bad mum for not even knowing what this stuff was for. I'm sure Nana didn't have them for me back in the eighties. I was feeling really overwhelmed, so I made a spreadsheet and prioritised the items. Top of the list was a pram. Even that turned out to be more complicated than I'd realised.

There aren't any UK manufacturers of triplet prams. The one that looked the best was made in New Zealand by a firm that had gone bust. Luckily, I tracked one down on eBay. When we went to pick it up and handed over £400 to a childminder in south-west London, the enormity of having triplets really hit.

We had a big car at the time, an Audi A4 estate. But we couldn't get the pram in. We were parked for about half an hour trying to work out how the hell to get it in the car, dismantling it and trying different angles. In the end, we had to fold down the back seats in order to make it work, and even then, it was tight!

There have been so many moments where we realised that what works for most normal families is just never going to work for us, but this was a big one. We would never be able to fit babies and the pram in the car. We would not be able to bring you home from hospital in this car. That is why we now have a purple campervan: three adults, three babies, our dog and the pram can fit comfortably!

We were given so much stuff by twin mums. I remember sorting through sacks of baby clothes and piling them up into different sizes. I held them up and thought how amazing and incredible it was that my babies would fit in these tiny vests. They looked like doll's clothes. Holding the clothes, it all felt really real. That these teeny, soft preemie babygrows would envelop your tiny, precious bodies. I gave those clothes a cuddle.

41

Even when I had to call an ambulance when I started to haemorrhage at home when I was 27 weeks pregnant, I couldn't allow myself to consider anything other than a happy ending for us all. I don't think my faith has ever been tested so much. As soon as I got to the hospital, they scanned me, and a very handsome Greek doctor reassured me you were all oblivious to me losing blood and chunks of placenta.

You're tough. I knew that. I knew you'd be absolute warriors in NICU and you were. I can't explain how unwhole I felt when you were no longer inside me but in incubators in a different part of the hospital. It was all so wrong. The mummies next to me and around me had their babies, and you were so far away. At this point, I couldn't even make it to the bathroom on my own, so you might as well have been on the moon.

Getting you well enough to come home was a mission. Saying goodbye to you every day and promising I'd be back soon broke my heart. Seeing you so fragile, so not ready to be here, so dependent on all the wires and machines was a trauma that took your dad and me a long, long time to process.

Yet we made it.

When you first got home, we were so out of our depth. We were doing 24 feeds every 24 hours! Your dad and I were so tired that we didn't even know if it was day or night. We set up a big cot for you to share and a changing table downstairs for daytime naps and changes, and put a massive cot bed right next to my bed because I wanted to be right next to you after all that separation. I didn't even mind when you fell asleep on me, not in your cot. I loved it.

Thank you for choosing me. For coming to me with divine timing. For showing me what's possible. For changing my life. For teaching me what really matters and reminding me how strong I am.

Dear Minnie

I'm welling up, so I'll stop writing now.

You know I've loved you since before you were here, and I will love you forever.

Mummy xxx

***

I CAN'T POSSIBLY COMPARE MY pregnancy to Leila's, but thinking back, lots of people are very gushy about the beauty of being pregnant, and of course, it is beautiful and a gift, but I can't say I floated through the entire nine months. For the first few months, I was sick every day. I was always sick in the mornings. I hadn't told loads of people that I was pregnant, but I remember I was filming *Sleeps Over* in America, and I was staying on people's sofas. The whole premise is that I was staying at people's houses, so I would get up and go for a walk in the garden and throw up. But no one knew apart from the boss (who I had to tell for insurance purposes!). Everyone was probably wondering why I kept sneaking off to the garden every morning! There was one family who were living in a trailer, and the air conditioning wasn't working. It was 40-odd degrees. I was lying in that trailer thinking, 'I can't possibly have anything else to throw up!' Luckily, from about five months onwards, I felt so much better.

I started to properly show when I was about six months, I reckon, and I liked showing my bump off. I enjoyed dressing when I was pregnant because it was unknown territory, and I wanted to celebrate my bump. It was only really near the end that I felt uncomfortable. I worked until I was eight and a half months pregnant, and I was filming with

43

Ukrainian civilians who were training with British soldiers to fight Russia. We were based at one of their northern base camps and were up and down mountains. It was snowing really heavily, and I was dodging grenades. I was wishing I could move a bit faster! The men were chivalrous, helped me over gates, and all wished me luck.

So talking to Leila about her triplet pregnancy was fascinating. After being pregnant with Minnie, I simply cannot imagine being pregnant with three babies at the same time.

Leila told me about the sheer physical effort of her pregnancy. 'I remember thinking, like an announcement on the train, that "all services are disrupted" was apt because it affected all parts of my body. I found that bits of my body that do their thing just stopped working, or weird stuff started happening because all my resources were being channelled towards these three growing babies. My gums and teeth got weak, and I ended up with eczema on my foot – different, weird things. I had nosebleeds and reflux. I got cramps, which would come on during the night and be incredibly painful.

'Normally, I am a fit person who does gym classes and runs upstairs, but I was massive, and my heart rate was high. I was like a beached whale and could not get off the sofa without someone helping me. I was this enormous weight. One of my boys – the singleton – was right in my ribs, so my ribs were pushing outwards, which was painful, and my two identical twins were lower down in the pelvic girdle area where you would expect a baby to be, but it was like being stretched from the inside out.'

According to the Twins Trust, in the UK, approximately one in every 65 pregnancies results in a multiple birth. Over the past 20 years, there has been an upward trend in the number of multiple births, attributed to fertility treatments, improved survival rates of premature babies, and women starting their families later. However, the multiple birth rate is now slowing down, aligning with the singleton birth rate. Twins are much more common than triplets; in 2019, 9,656 sets of twins and 143 sets of triplets and above were born. There are also many more twins and triplets born due to IVF than naturally conceived pregnancies like Leila's. According to the same research, on average, 11 per cent of IVF pregnancies result in either twins or triplets, compared to 1–2 per cent of naturally conceived pregnancies. Multiple embryos are sometimes transferred during a cycle to save costs and increase the chances of success, especially if the couple is limited to just one IVF cycle on the NHS. However, according to the Human Fertilisation and Embryology Authority (HFEA), if you have multiple high-quality embryos available, the current best practice for most women is to transfer just one embryo into the womb and freeze the others – this is known as an elective single embryo transfer. This approach helps reduce the risk of multiple births, which can present serious health risks for both the mother and babies, including a higher likelihood of premature birth or low birth weight. In some cases, a clinic may determine that transferring more than one embryo is appropriate, particularly for older women who have a lower overall chance of success and are less likely to have two embryos implant successfully.

Leila was immaculately dressed and made-up and looked so together for someone with triplet toddlers at home. Before she got pregnant, she ran a successful publishing company with her brother and was voted a top 100 female entrepreneur. For someone so clearly in control, I asked her if she could possibly have imagined what life would be like when her babies arrived.

'I remember saying to someone that it was like jumping off a cliff and having no idea what the thing you are going to land in is, because it is going to be so totally different,' she recalled in a no-nonsense way.

'I spoke to a few triplet mums to get an idea of what their lives were like and their experiences, but that was largely preparing me for the birth and hospital phase, when the babies would be in the neonatal hospital care unit, and how to deal with the medical stress with all of that, rather than it being what it was like to feed three babies a day.

'I did do a one-day event that the Twins Trust does to prepare you for parenthood, and I came away thinking, "How the F are we going to do this?" There is no way we can fit all the work we need to do in a day into a day. We were given a piece of paper with a list of jobs and how long each should take, and however we totted it up, we couldn't get to 24 hours, even when we were only giving ourselves four hours' sleep. We were the only triplet parents in that group; everyone else had twins, and that was a moment of feeling it would be impossible.'

Leila described the early days as 'chaos'.

'At the very beginning, the first week, we did not know if it was day or night, up or down. We did not know what was going on. It was so crazy; we couldn't understand how they could be discharged. There was a stressful energy to them. It was like they had been ripped out of the womb before they were ready. They weren't supposed to be here, and it wasn't right. As a mum, I was trying to make it right and give them what they needed. Over a few months, this eased, and we found a pattern and rhythm with it. I also had a maternity nurse who came a few weeks after they were born and helped set up proper bed and bath routines. Without her, I think that hot-mess phase would've rumbled on a lot longer.'

Leila says the newborn phase became easier when her babies were around three months old.

'At that point, the wake-up patterns became more predictable, and they would wake up at roughly the same times every night, and we would get the stretches of sleep between them,' she explained. 'In the beginning, it was a hot mess. They were waking up all over the show and waking each other up. They started to get less sensitive to the noise of the others, and that helped too, and we were more battle-hardy and knew what we were doing a bit more.'

When I spoke to Leila about being a mum of three, it was clear she is passionate about not feeling 'mum guilt'.

'I think I am different to other mums, and it is hard to articulate why that is, but I think, because of the intensity of having three, you have this very compressed period to get stuff done, especially in that newborn period, and it's just brutal. And if you've got that times three, you reach a kind of exhaustion point quite quickly. Wellness and self-care are not a nice-to-have; I knew that if I did not do it, then I would not survive. It's such an evolutionary fuck up that these babies could kill their mum before they were three months old! I needed to be sure that I could last the distance.'

Leila said she was quick to carve out some me-time. 'I had to really claim time for myself – to go to the gym and get out, because otherwise I just wouldn't have survived. So, I'm pro mums looking after themselves and not feeling guilty about it. It's the sustainability factor, and just burning out early doors is not going to help my children, it's not going to help my husband, who definitely can't step up and do what I do, and this whole family is going down unless I'm looking after myself.'

It's funny that Leila used the word 'sustainability', because it's something I would talk about in my early days as a mum. My experience is not comparable at all to Leila's, but I remember at one stage when the breast pump was broken, I was so knackered, I had been wearing the same outfit day after day and hadn't had a shower for a week; I said: 'This doesn't feel sustainable.' I remember telling Kev that it couldn't be that exhausting forever; there must be a moment when it would start to feel easier. Leila is right; the idea that you can soldier on and not wash or eat sounds ridiculous.

Leila added: 'I think you have to really fight to tell the people around you that you need a break.'

Just to add from my own perspective – people coming round so you can hoover; this is not a break.

My conversation with Leila reminded me of an article I read in the *New Yorker* about mums in Taipei, in Taiwan, who are invited to a postpartum centre for a month. These places have nurses, amazing food and a fluffy bed to hang out in. New mums have the option to reside in one of about 280 designated hotels. During their stay, they will enjoy meals, 24/7 childcare, medical consultations, and extra benefits like yoga sessions and breastfeeding support. It's a totally different take on our attitudes in the West. Here, we get to come home, have a handful of medical checks, and that's it. For mums like Leila, advice like 'sleeping when the baby sleeps' was not helpful as, unsurprisingly, her newborn triplets were rarely all asleep at the same time.

Leila adds: 'I've always been very capable. I think when you are mentally capable, people don't offer help, because obviously, I'm not someone who's traditionally very good at asking for help. And so they just see me, and I look like I'm on top of everything, but it would be so great if someone asked: "Can I get you a cup of coffee?"'

I think many mums can battle a bit with the idea of doing stuff for themselves. In my mind, I feel I can justify being away from Minnie if I'm working, but if I have an hour or two free to do my hair or nails, I do find myself feeling a bit guilty and sometimes, in those moments, the idea that I should be with her can linger. And I know it's daft. When I'm not working, I'm hanging out with her all the time. Logically, I know I also want to do nice shit for myself. It's important for so many reasons to prioritise yourself, but yes, I can see how we also find it tricky. Prioritising our own well-being surely improves our relationships with our children. When we are happier and more balanced, we all benefit. So, my public service announcement: get that blow-dry and book those shellacs!

4

'I am part of a club no one wants to belong to.'

A story of loss

Dear Gabe,

I'll always smile when I remember the moment I found out you were coming to join our family. From the second I saw both lines on the pregnancy test, you were instantly loved. It was the start of a new year, a year that would become life-changing.

In those early weeks of pregnancy, despite how tired I felt and the nausea I experienced, I immediately felt we were a team. Do you remember our adventures? Hikes in the hills above Marsden, dips at the local swimming pool and even when you very kindly settled my nerves by accompanying me to a job interview. I was so excited and looked forward to a lifetime of showing you the world.

At the first ultrasound scan, your lively and perhaps a little rebellious character shone through on the screen, and hearing your heartbeat was a dream come true. I was already a proud mum and stared for hours at the scan pictures I was handed, counting down until the next time I would get to see you.

However, weeks later, my deep joy turned to deep sorrow when, at the next appointment, the room turned quiet. The doctors' faces looked concerned, and it felt like I'd fallen through a trapdoor when I found out how poorly you were. You had all the markers for a rare but very severe genetic condition called Edwards' syndrome (T18), and you had the most serious form of it. Together with your daddy, I sought further medical advice, screenings and second opinions, fighting as hard as I could to protect you and keep you safe. But as the days and weeks passed, it became clear that, tragically, you wouldn't ever be well enough to come home with me.

The 'decision' – and I say decision lightly, as the word feels insufficient – to say goodbye to you was made with the most love but the biggest heartbreak. If love could have saved you, my boy, you would have lived forever.

I remember that March day like it was yesterday, welcoming you into the world at the hospital; you were small, but gosh, you were perfect, with ten tiny fingers and ten tiny toes. I studied every part of you. Saying both hello and goodbye on the same day was one of the hardest things I have ever had to do.

You were named Gabriel, or Gabe for short (I hope you like it), and not a single day has passed without you being in my thoughts or my saying your name. It's actually your birthday soon, and I'm thinking about another fun way to mark it this year.

Despite you not making it home with me and even though it's hard sometimes, when in the eyes of some, I may sadly not appear to be a mother, never forget, Gabe, that I will forever identify as your mum; you will always be a huge part of my life.

My journey into motherhood may be outwardly less visible to others, but it's no less of a journey than if you were here in my arms. In fact, it's because of you that I have found and connected with many other parents throughout the UK and even across the globe, all of whom, just like me, are navigating life after baby loss . . . It's a club none of us wanted a lifetime membership to, but it's without doubt full of the very best members, many of whom I'm now grateful to call friends . . . my 'mum friends'. It's been many of these surprising new connections that have really helped me make sense of this new life path I'm on, and I have you to thank for bringing all of these kind souls into my life.

I love talking about you and finding new ways to keep you present and your memory alive; I never want it to dim. You really are my motivation in all that I do. I will continue to make sure you see the world through my eyes, and I hope you enjoy it.

I will always be grateful for the fresh perspective you gave me on life and can say with certainty that carrying you for all your life was my greatest honour. Thanks for choosing me to be your mum.

So, until we meet again, son . . . don't get into too much mischief with your little pals wherever you all are.

Love Mum x

***

WHEN I FIRST THOUGHT ABOUT motherhood, I felt it was important to hear from someone who didn't have her baby at home with her. When you are pregnant, you are aware that you are housing your baby. The main objective is to make sure it all goes well, and then you meet your baby. That is the dream, so I can't imagine – and how could any of us who haven't had that experience – what it must feel like when things go wrong.

According to the NHS, miscarriages, occurring before 24 weeks of pregnancy, are estimated to happen in one in eight known pregnancies, though the rate might be higher when including pregnancies that end before a woman even knows she's pregnant. Stillbirths are defined as the loss of a baby at or after 24 weeks. In England, approximately 1 in 250 births results in a stillbirth.

'There are lots and lots of people who might have different experiences of being mums that are not necessarily as visible as everyone else's,' Clare told me. 'There are so many different ways that you can end up being like this; heartbreaking ways that mean your baby does not come home.'

Clare describes her experience as being 'part of a club that no one wants to be a member of'.

It must be unimaginably tough to try and navigate that experience and tell people what has happened while grieving yourself. I asked Clare whether she sought support, and she found a group for TFMR mums (women who have had 'terminations for medical reasons'). This could be due to a serious chromosomal, genetic or structural fetal abnormality, or a situation where continuing the pregnancy would risk the health or life of the mother. According to Tommy's in 2020, at least 5,000 pregnancies a year end in TFMR, but often people find it hard to discuss it, and it is rarely spoken about.

Charities, including Tommy's, ARC and Petals, believe that the secrecy surrounding TFMR can leave people to navigate this traumatic experience in isolation, which can severely impact their mental health. They explain that people in this situation can find it hard to seek out the right support due to the complicated feelings they have around making this decision and fearing others judging them for it.

'I found an online support group for mums in my situation. It had just started a few months earlier,' Clare explained. 'So when I joined them, there were about two or three hundred people. Now there are thousands all over the world. The lady who runs it is a lifesaver. She pulled together various resources and put on Zoom support meetings. Everybody just got it, with zero judgement, because we all felt similar emotions of grief but also sometimes guilt, linked to having had to make the decision to say goodbye. Did you do enough? Could we have done something different?

'I connected with a lot of the people that I speak to regularly through this group, and I've met many people online and in person. I made a friend, Lucy, who literally lives around the corner from me. I ended up meeting with her, and we believe that her son, Oscar, and Gabe are good friends. It might sound crazy, but we believe they are out there some-where making mischief.'

Clare spoke about her determination that Gabe somehow lives on through her. 'I love his name, and I can hear myself saying that name for the rest of my life. It just felt so right. And when everyone says, "Oh, so he must be really angelic?" I say, "No, I'm absolutely convinced he is a rascal."

'I'm not religious. I don't necessarily believe in heaven, and I don't believe he's up there in the clouds. But if he were, I have a feeling he'd be with a catapult, trying to get some good shots!'

We talked about the emotions associated with the anniversaries of certain events and how hard they might be for mothers like her.

'It was his birthday yesterday,' Clare told me quietly. 'I find that the build-up to those days is always worse. I found last week [emotionally] quite heavy. Then, on the day, I normally feel quite calm. My partner and I went on a bike ride and had a little cake for him. I really feel quite strongly that if he is watching somewhere with his pals, I want him to look down and think: "That's my folks doing something fun." I want to give him an interesting life to watch. I believe that when I explore new places, he sees them through my eyes.'

It was interesting to hear how Gabe has shaped Clare's identity. It goes without saying that anyone who hasn't had to face a similar situation can't even begin to understand what it's like. Only those who have been through this kind of loss will ever truly get it. It made me think about the ways we grieve and how for mothers who never get to take their babies home – whether due to miscarriage, TFMR, stillbirth or other reasons – this must be a particularly heartbreaking process. Listening back to our chat reminded me of an article I read in *The New York Times* about a lovely ritual in Japan. Babies are represented with Jizo figurines, small stone statues dressed in bibs and caps, which in Buddhist teachings honour the souls of babies who are never born. The Jizo serves a dual purpose; the image represents both the soul of the deceased infant or fetus and the deity who cares for children on their journey in the other world. These figurines sit in Japanese cemeteries and offer parents a way to express their love, and some leave toys, flowers and snacks for their children in the afterlife.

Clare and I also talked at length about how to navigate the seemingly innocent question, 'Do you have kids?' This question is often part of everyday small talk when you meet new people. But for so many people, for many, many different reasons, the answer is not that simple.

'Sometimes the easy answer is just to say no,' Clare explained, carefully. 'It's just easier, but it really doesn't sit well to say that because I feel like I'm doing Gabe a disservice.

'You have to really judge quickly to work out if you feel OK to share that information with the person and if you've time to explain. If it's a quick, fleeting conversation, it's not the right moment to say you do have a son, and he's just not at home. If you start that conversation and you don't get a chance to finish it properly, it can make the other person feel terrible.'

We talked about some of the right questions to ask, which are more open-ended and inclusive.

'I would just ask people, "Tell me about your family," because that's so open-ended. You can talk about your partner, dog, or whatever. As a society, we are obsessed with asking people about kids, and maybe – like me – it's a different outcome.'

5

'It felt like especially precious cargo.'

A story of surrogacy

Dear Bea and Robin,

This letter is all about what led me to your parents and then, incredibly, you.

After a really difficult time in 2009 with the loss of our first baby, I never thought I would become a mummy to three gorgeous children. My younger sister was really struggling to conceive, and the thought crossed my mind – could I help her? Thankfully, she ended up falling pregnant and now has two boys. I was overjoyed for her, but the feeling of being able to help never left me. After the birth of my youngest, I felt compelled to look into egg donation.

In 2017, I donated my eggs to a couple who couldn't have children. They, like my sister, had struggled for years to have a baby. I was matched with them via an organisation. In 2017, they had a little girl, and in 2020, they had twin girls. The joy I felt when I found out they were pregnant was incredible. I felt so proud to have contributed to them becoming parents. However, I did often wonder who the couple were and what their daughters were like: what their personalities were like, what they looked like and if they had my curly hair! In the future, I hope they reach out if they want to know me and find out more about their genetic history.

During 2017, I met a friend through donating my eggs who told me about an organisation called Surrogacy UK. I was told you would meet intended parents organically and the ethos is all built on friendship. I liked the sound of that! My husband and I initially joined as a 'known egg donor', but after the Surrogacy UK annual conference, we soon changed our minds. We met so many incredible people that we just knew, we had to help. The weekend was filled with sessions for surrogates and their partners and we learnt so much from people who had been in the organisation for years. It felt like a community of like-minded people who just wanted to help. In the evening they had a quiz and a disco and we met your parents, Bea. When the evening event had finished, my husband said to me, 'We have to do this, don't we? If we would help our family, why wouldn't we help people that become family?' This is how Surrogacy UK felt and still feels; like we were with family.

We met both your parents through this organisation, and it has utterly changed our lives. It has enriched our lives in so many ways. Our children were seven, five and two when we joined, and they are now 13, 11 and 8. It has taught us all about kindness, compassion, patience, understanding and happiness beyond belief. The friendship we made with your parents was the start of something so special. The friendship we have with both your parents is more than just surrogacy; it is a relationship that transcends it. I will have always carried you, and surrogacy is part of your story, but you're so much more than that. We want to meet up with you all because we love you and your parents.

The day I gave birth to you, Bea, was so warm, and I was five days overdue. It was the middle of lockdown, but we were so lucky to have a water birth at home. I remember you being born into your mummy's arms with your daddy watching. As I turned around, I watched all that heartache ease, and they instantly fell in love. You were finally here. I also knew, in that moment, that if I could help another family, I would.

Robin, the day you were born was so magical, and after the birth, I watched your mummy and daddy hold you with a look of pure joy on their faces. Their decade of trying to become parents was finally over. We all spent 12 hours together in the delivery room and it was a privilege watching them get to know you.

I feel so honoured to have carried you both for nine months and delivered you safely into the arms of your parents. They say the best thing you can ever do is become a parent. Watching your parents fall in love with you in front of my eyes will be the next best thing. They looked like they were at peace. Completely overwhelmed and completely in love. We love seeing you with your parents and we try to meet up every few months. I am honoured to be your godmother, Bea, and I love how I will always be in both your lives.

You will both be two of the most wonderful things I have ever been part of, and I can't wait to watch you grow in this crazy journey of life.

All my love,

Auntie Rena

***

I REALLY BELIEVE THAT SURROGACY is an incredibly selfless act. I find this topic fascinating, particularly now that I am a mother. I have interviewed surrogates as part of my TV work, but Rena was the first surrogate I spoke to since having Minnie. I can't imagine being able to want to help someone or a family so much that I would be able to do this.

When I told her this, Rena explained: 'I don't think I would've contemplated being a surrogate if I didn't already have my family. I knew our family was complete when we started on this journey.

'When I first mentioned surrogacy to my husband, I think he thought I was off my rocker. I was just a few months ahead of him. When we went to the conference, it all fell into place for him. He's been incredible. I'm too old to do it again – I think I would fall apart, but I have loved it.'

I asked Rena whether, when she was carrying her surrogate babies, she felt like she acted differently – either consciously or subconsciously – and whether they felt like different pregnancies to the ones she had with her own babies.

'Yes, they felt like entirely different pregnancies, and it's all to do with the mindset,' she explained. 'From the point of conception, I know they are never mine. It also felt like there was a lot more responsibility. It sounds awful, and it's not that I wasn't careful when I was carrying my own kids, but with my surrogate babies, it felt like especially precious cargo. There is definitely a bond, and I love the two babies I carried, but it is not a maternal love – I feel like more of an aunty figure.'

She said that recovery after birth was 'a dream'.

'I woke up to messages in the morning after a beautiful night's sleep, saying, "You never told me that they wake up every hour!" But the recovery was much easier. I think the issue was more that I forgot that I had had a baby because they were not with me. You do forget.'

Surrogacy in the UK is different from other countries, including the US. I met a potential surrogate in the US who was going to help a couple where there was an age gap. The male partner was significantly younger than his partner, who already had children. They were looking to start a family and needed assistance, but the difference was that they could pay her. In the UK, commercial surrogacy is prohibited, and only altruistic arrangements are permitted, where the surrogate receives only 'reasonable expenses', which might include living expenses like maternity clothing, medical costs or compensation for time off work. Legal parenthood is determined by the birth certificate, requiring a court order for the intended parents to become legal parents. In the UK, the laws surrounding it were made in the eighties. Surrogacy agreements are not enforceable by law, so clear communication and trust are essential from the outset. Regardless of the laws and situation, I think, with all the surrogate women I have met, there is an innate desire to help others have a family. I was interested to read figures in a report from the University of Kent and My Surrogacy Journey, a non-profit organisation which supports surrogates and intended parents, which showed that the number of parents using a surrogate to have a family in England and Wales had quadrupled in a decade. In 2011, there were 117 parental orders, transferring legal parentage from the surrogate, and in 2020 there were 413.

Rena told me about the support she had from the organisation Surrogacy UK and the fact that surrogacies had to be built on friendship from the start.

'We built such a beautiful bond,' she told me. 'We are friends for life. I knew that both sets of couples were on my side, fighting my corner. You spend a long time getting to know them, and it has to be the right team for you. We always say in surrogacy that you need to find your tribe.'

Surrogacy can involve using the surrogate's own eggs, while gestational surrogacy uses the intended mother's eggs or those from a donor.

When I asked Rena about the more challenging parts of surrogacy, she explained that her first couple lost their last embryos.

'It can be very hard when it doesn't go to plan,' she said. 'With our first couple, the mother knew from a very young age that she wouldn't be able to carry herself and had looked into surrogacy for a number of years. She did have embryos, so it was particularly hard when I lost them. To have to tell your friend that you are having a miscarriage and losing their baby is a whole other level of hard. I felt like I had failed her.

'She kept saying to me, "I know you have done everything you can," but it was horrible. That's when I offered to use my eggs. I went into gestational surrogacy naively thinking that I am fertile, with three of my own kids when, actually, that doesn't mean anything. It's the viability of the embryo that is the most important thing when it comes to a successful pregnancy. So, there can be lots of lows and lots of unbelievable highs.'

Rena's surrogate baby, Bea, is genetically related to her, but she says that to her, genetics means very little.

'I have learnt so much. She will always be genetically related to me and have genetic siblings, but I am not her mum. Her mum is the person who has brought her up and looked after her from the moment she was born. To me, that is love; it's not about genetics.'

Rena told me how being a surrogate has profoundly changed her life. 'When I first started thinking about surrogacy, I thought I would do something kind to help and then go on my merry way.

'I had no idea how much we would all gain from it. It's taught my children so much about being understanding. You never know what people are going through, which has made them think about things differently. We call surrogacy "extreme babysitting".'

Her only regret? 'I wish I had started a bit younger. I would have loved to continue to help if I could.'

6

'Who gets the opportunity to go on maternity leave together?'

A story of shared motherhood

Dear Ezra and Elvis,

What a wild IVF journey we have had . . . That led us to you. Our little miracles born just eight weeks apart.

We are the first couple to have this procedure – known as simultaneous reciprocal IVF – in the UK. See – making firsts already! Reciprocal IVF is sometimes called shared motherhood. This means that eggs are collected from one partner and fertilised using donor sperm. The most viable embryos are then selected for transfer into the other partner's uterus to start the pregnancy.

We always thought it would be a lush thing to do – to carry each other's babies. We never knew it was an actual 'thing' until a friend carried her partner's baby. We both felt it would be amazing to have twins, and this was a special way to do it. Both of us have quite a large gap between us and our siblings. We wanted you two to be close in age and grow up together, play together and be each other's biggest champions. We also thought it would be a special way of feeling connected to you both.

When we came to choosing our donor, there was no great ceremony. It was a Thursday night, and we started swiping through sperm banks. We chose a man about our own age who had two children and was donating for altruistic reasons – his family was struggling with infertility, and he wanted to help others.

We built an amazing community online. With IVF, there was a lot of waiting, anticipation and anxiety. As we went through each stage, we felt the next one would be easier, but it never was – it just opened the door to more uncertainty. It was a rollercoaster of a process.

Our pregnancies were quite different, a bit yin and yang. Elvis, you made your impression from the start! You made Mummy Emily look a bit like a moose; I was so swollen and fat. Comparatively, Mummy Kerry's pregnancy with you, Ezra, was a breeze. Because of this, we were convinced you were different sexes, but we were so shocked and felt like we had hit the jackpot when we discovered you were both boys. Most of all, though, being pregnant together was fun and helped us really understand what the other was going through.

Now that we have had you, we feel an incredible connection to you both in different ways. Kerry gave birth to you, Ezra, and Emily gave birth to you, Elvis. We expected you both to look like the donor, as we have seen a picture of him as a child, simply because you were boys, but you look just like us. Ezra, you have amazing ginger hair like Emily's grandad, and Elvis, you have Kerry's button nose and big eyes. As we are writing, you are just a few weeks old, but your personalities are shining through already.

Dear Minnie

We feel connected like a unique puzzle with four corners and every piece in place. We have both found a whole different level of love, like a new chamber in our hearts for our babies.

Life feels quite crazy now — a shower or even having a poo feels like a luxury. Our lives were changed in a split second by you two, but we have never felt love like it. There is nothing better than the way you look at us.

We are beyond grateful for the magic of science, and we are so excited about our future with you. We can't wait to spend the rest of our lives making you as happy as you make us.

Love,

Mummy Emily & Mummy Kerry

***

It was emily who first came up with the idea of having babies at the same time through reciprocal IVF. Reciprocal IVF, also known as co-maternity or co-IVF, is a distinctive assisted reproductive technology (ART) that allows both partners to be involved in the conception and pregnancy process. This method enables both parents to play a significant role in creating and nurturing their child. In reciprocal IVF, one partner undergoes ovarian stimulation and has her eggs retrieved. These eggs are then fertilised with donor sperm to form embryos. One of these embryos is subsequently transferred into the uterus of the other partner. This process allows one partner to provide the genetic material, while the other offers the nurturing environment for the pregnancy,

69

enabling both to have a significant role in the development of the fetus and child. In this case, they did the procedure at the same time, so an embryo created from Emily's egg was implanted in Kerry, and vice versa, so they were carrying each other's biological children. It was the first time this procedure had been attempted in the UK.

Kerry had always been more maternal, while Emily hadn't considered it until they were together. During the extended hours of lockdown, they talked about their future and decided they wanted to create a family where they could both be biological and gestational mothers.

Kerry recalled in a matter-of-fact tone: 'There was no great ceremony, it was a Thursday night, and we started swiping through sperm banks. The problem is that once you start, you can't stop, there is so much choice. We chose a man about the same age as us, who already had kids. He was donating out of a desire to help others because some of his family members were also struggling with infertility.'

Even though they underwent similar procedures at the same time, both women explained they were open-minded that IVF could work for one of them and not the other.

Emily said: 'We knew one of us might be waiting for weeks, months or years, and it might never happen.'

Kerry added: 'We hadn't had a scan or anything before that point [when we started treatment], but we keep recommending it to people now. It's something that would be really good for couples who aren't planning to have children until their late thirties. You certainly don't want to get to that point and find out it's more difficult.'

Emily fell pregnant after her first attempt, but Kerry had to go another round to succeed.

They also spoke about the issues of having IVF while working – Kerry is a teacher, and Emily is a producer.

'It's really, really tough to be going through IVF when you're working: you don't want to tell anyone because that adds pressure to the situation,' Emily added. 'And if you're not having IVF, you might say to your friends that you are trying for a baby, but you don't announce it the day after having sex.

'Going through IVF as a heterosexual or same-sex couple, you need lots of time off for appointments, basically to potentially get pregnant. There are working guidelines about having reasonable time off for medical reasons, but with IVF, you need so much time off. It's quite a private thing as well.'

Kerry added, 'It's hard enough going through the IVF process, let alone having to navigate getting time off. In my job as a teacher, I don't get time off outside the holidays. So I tried to plan appointments within the holidays, but you have to change tack when certain things don't work out.'

Kerry told me that when they shared the news with friends and family that they were both pregnant, some people around them were worried about certain aspects of being pregnant at the same time.

'They asked us questions like, "Who's going to pick up after the dog? What if you go into labour at the same time?" There was a small chance of that, but hopefully, it wouldn't happen.'

Emily added: 'The first thing that surprised us was that being pregnant together was fine. I think unless you've been pregnant, you wouldn't really understand some of the things that a pregnant person goes through. It was great that we could empathise with each other and how the other was feeling. We wanted to look after each other. We didn't know anything different because neither of us had ever been pregnant before. But we also knew we had to carry on.'

When I met them, Elvis was having a nap and Ezra was feeding and they were still in the throes of the early days of motherhood. Emily laughed as she described it as 'being kicked repeatedly in the fanny'.

'We feel like we are keeping our chin above water. But we are starting to be more mindful about looking after ourselves. Even just having a shower can make you feel so much better.'

They were keen that people be 'more honest about the hard bits. We think it's just like people don't talk about it – being so tired you want to crawl into a hole.'

Emily gave birth to Elvis on New Year's Day, while Ezra arrived a few weeks later after an emergency caesarean.

Kerry described watching Emily giving birth as a 'massacre'.

'Watching her give birth was a bit like a massacre and very emotional, and I knew I would have to give birth too a few weeks later. My friends told me Ezra would just fall out, but it was not like that at all because I had an emergency C-section.'

I also had a C-section with Minnie. She was upside down. The doctor told me there were various options, including trying to manually turn her round, but in the end we went with the planned caesarean. On reflection, it was pretty plain sailing, really – which I know is such a luxury. I hear of so many people who have just the most difficult or frightening labour, and I always think about how terrifying that must be, especially when you're already feeling so exposed and vulnerable. Mums really are unbelievable! On the day of the caesarean, I went in first thing in the morning, was given my compression stockings and gown and sat there in the waiting room with a bunch of other women. I remember feeling starving. And thirsty. It's all just so, so surreal! The night before I barely slept – it was like, 'So what, tomorrow I'm going to have a baby?!' I obviously was apprehensive but I wouldn't say I was riddled with nerves. (That came later, when I was sat on the hospital bed waiting to be wheeled into theatre!) I kept telling myself that so many women have babies, and I started thinking of all the women I know who are mothers, and surely if it were that horrific they wouldn't go on to do it again?!

It felt like it must be doable.

Kev told me that the night before he had sat in the car and prayed out loud that we would both be OK.

Reflecting on my birth to Emily and Kerry, I remembered how hilarious the whole thing was. I was WAY more dramatic than I had anticipated. I mean, generally, I would describe myself as quite pragmatic and level-headed, but that went out the WINDOW when I was lying on that bed. When they gave me that epidural, I could feel it rising up my body, and I'd convinced myself I couldn't breathe. I remember the anaesthetist telling me, 'Your oxygen levels are 100 per cent.' Kev jokes that halfway through I was trying to make a run for it, off the bed and into the corridor. Don't ask me what on earth I was thinking, because I couldn't move my fucking legs! Ridiculous!

'I had no idea recovery after a C-section would be so hard,' Kerry said. 'I was like a slug for weeks, trying to move. Sitting up took me a long time! I moved like a demented mermaid.'

One of the things I remember most clearly after having Minnie is just never letting go of the baby when I was in the hospital. I was lying there, high on loads of drugs for a couple of days. Leaving the hospital, it was like two idiots trying to parent – we didn't have a clue what we were doing. We couldn't get Minnie into the car seat, and the midwives were so sweet and trying to help us strap her in. When we got in the car, my boobs were leaking, I was obsessed with the car being the right temperature (too hot, too cold, just right? If the windows are down, is it too fumey?). Kev was driving really carefully across London, but every time we hit a speed bump, I was in agony. I didn't realise the pain would be so bad.

If there had been cameras in our house that first night we brought Minnie home, it would've been a smash-hit comedy series; it was such a saga. The pair of us were running around like headless chickens, naked, with no idea what we were doing. Love her heart – Minnie must've been looking at the pair of us, thinking: 'Who on earth have they sent me to – are these my parents?!'

We talked about sleep deprivation in the early days almost killing most mums. And then, just at the point when you are having an existential crisis, they get to six weeks and start to smile. It's as if you're running an ultramarathon, and just at the moment when you have nothing left, that smile arrives and pushes you over the line.

Despite their bleary-eyed tiredness, I loved talking with Kerry and Emily. They seemed to spark off each other's energy; they are clearly a dynamic parenting team.

When I asked them about people's reactions, the mums said that when they are out and about and meeting new people, the reaction to them has been overwhelmingly positive.

Emily said: 'When we're walking down the street, people like to be nosey because we've got a double buggy. So, they're like, "Oh, twins!"

Obviously, Elvis is two months older than Ezra and much bigger. As we explain, seeing people's faces as they try to work it out is fun.

'You get some people who really get it – it's usually the younger people who are more accepting. Some older people don't really get it – you can see them rolling into an early grave. But overall, the general consensus has been amazing.'

They told me about how they are really excited about the future, including a trip they were planning to Southeast Asia and New Zealand during their maternity leaves.

Kerry said: 'The one thing that we said before we had the boys was we don't want our life to change too much because we have a lot of things that we still want to do, mainly travelling. Who gets the opportunity to go on maternity leave together?'

They also talked about the simple things they can't wait to do with their boys.

'Our lives have changed dramatically. We are just showing them what life is all about. And there's so much to look forward to.'

Part II
Birth

7

'You were and will always be the best surprise we'll ever have.'

A story of teenage motherhood

Dear Alexis,

When you were born, I was only 16. I'd just finished my GCSEs and was getting ready to celebrate prom with all my friends. Your arrival came very much as a surprise, and unlike most, I didn't have the time to prepare for your arrival, as I didn't know I was pregnant.

On the day you were born, I spent the day helping your dad get his suit ready for prom and doing last-minute preparations, like painting my nails and practising how I was going to do my make-up. We were really excited about prom; we had worked so hard and were just ready to let our hair down and celebrate with all our friends.

Dad and I had been together for about three years. I can't really remember what I liked about your dad; I just remember saying to a friend at youth club that I thought he was attractive. The next minute, we were boyfriend and girlfriend – we hadn't even had a conversation! Apart from a few childhood boyfriends, Dad was and will always be the love of my life. (I know when you read this, you'll cringe, but I only wish the same for you one day!)

I felt strange all day. I knew my period was due, and they'd been regular every month, so I didn't think much of it. As the day went on, the pain got worse. It began as an achy pain in my back, but it later felt more like a stabbing pain that seemed to come and go every 20 minutes or so. I couldn't eat and just took myself straight to bed. I tossed and turned. I couldn't get comfortable.

Eventually, after what felt like hours, I decided to go to the toilet to see if that would help. I sat in the bathroom for about half an hour when all of a sudden, a gush of water came. I had no idea what was happening, and panic started to set in, but I was too scared to call for help. I had this natural urge to push, and that's when your head started to appear. I still wasn't 100 per cent sure at this point what was happening, but then it clicked: 'I'm having a baby!' It was weird; as soon as I knew what was happening, I knew I needed to keep pushing to ensure nothing happened to you. I pulled you out myself and just stared down at you, thinking, 'Oh my God, what do I do now?'

Thinking back, it still doesn't feel real, and I ask myself, 'How did I do that?'

I snapped back to reality when your uncle tried to come to the toilet! I screamed at him to get Nanna, and the rest was a bit of a blur. I remember Nanna seeing you for the first time; she was very pale and could barely speak, but she very quickly went into 'mum mode'. She grabbed towels to keep you warm and helped me out of the bathroom. She made Pops call for an ambulance – she just knew what to do. The face of the paramedic when he was told we didn't know you were coming will always make me laugh. His jaw dropped, he stumbled over his words and just didn't know what to say, bless him! He was stunned. He eventually called out more paramedics, who were also just as shocked as he that I didn't know I was pregnant. They were a little worried about your temperature, so they put you in a warm sheet and stuffed you down Nanna's jumper, then blue-lighted us to Poole hospital. You were taken straight to NICU to be checked over and monitored whilst I had tests done myself.

None of the nurses could quite believe the story, so I had a lot of visitors asking me lots of questions! They asked me a lot, but a nurse asked one question that stood out. She asked, 'Do you want to keep her?'

Thinking back, the question wasn't as blunt as that, but in so many words, this is what she was asking me. She appreciated that I'd been through a lot, but I'd not planned for any of this to happen. I fully understood why she needed to ask. I didn't even have to think: regardless of having no time to prepare for you, you were my little girl, and I was going to care for you as best I could. As soon as I saw you, I fell in love instantly. I completely forgot I was a 16-year-old. I knew I had to become a mum, and that was the best feeling. Dad felt the same and that was it. Dad found out about you by a phone call from Nanna on our way to the hospital. He was definitely shocked, but he was just worried about us and wanted to make sure we were both OK. I showered and was moved up to a private room where Nanna could stay with me whilst you spent the first night in NICU. Dad went home to help get things prepared and just take in your arrival before we brought you home. I couldn't sleep; I was eager to see you properly and give you your first feed.

Later the following day, we were both moved to the maternity ward, where we spent our first night together without any family to help. I cried when Nanna had to leave. I knew I was in the best place if I needed help with you, but I think I was worried I wouldn't be able to cope without Nanna there. I wasn't alone, but I felt alone. But a lovely midwife took care of us and made me feel at ease. She helped with night feeds, as she could see I was exhausted, and helped when we needed. I only needed her help when you had a poo explosion, and I needed another pair of hands!

On the third day, it was finally time to take you home. I was excited, nervous, scared, but I just wanted to get you home. We got back to a lounge full of baby stuff. Friends and family had brought over bouncy chairs, clothes, everything I obviously didn't have. I felt truly overwhelmed, loved and happy that everyone accepted their new life with you in it. The next couple of days were just about getting into a routine and introducing you to family and friends. When friends visited and heard the story, they couldn't quite believe it! But they didn't let it change anything. We carried on going for coffee and dinner dates; you just tagged along! They were as helpful as they could be and so supportive. Everyone was shocked and had a million questions, but ultimately they were happy for us, and were always there if we needed them.

We had the summer to enjoy getting used to our new life as a family of three and adjusting to being teen parents. After the summer, Dad and I both decided to go to college/sixth form to try and get a further education so we could do our best to provide for you later in life. We got part-time jobs to make sure we could still do fun things with you on the weekends. And the rest is history. I cannot imagine life without you now. You've taught me so much and helped me become the person I am today.

You are now eight, and Dad and I are married. You were our beautiful little flower girl; having you as part of our day was amazing. We've loved watching you grow into the little madam you are today! You were and will always be the best surprise we'll ever have.

Love Mum x

***

W HEN I HEARD KAITLIN'S STORY, I was amazed. But everything about her experience is incredible and a testament to her and her husband.

'It's crazy looking back and to see where we are now,' Kaitlin said. 'Telling new people is quite funny to see their reaction.'

Kaitlin explained that she was doing GCSE dance, and the practical exam had finished a lot earlier in the year, so she had started to put on a bit of weight but definitely did not look – or feel – pregnant. Her menstrual cycle was regular.

'There was no indication that I was pregnant,' Kaitlin explained.

Kaitlin had a cryptic pregnancy, sometimes called a hidden or stealth pregnancy, and it is more common than you might think. A 2002 study published in the *British Medical Journal* estimated that it occurs in approximately 1 in every 2,500 pregnancies, indicating roughly 320 cases annually in the UK. Although research is limited – likely due to the surprising nature of the condition – cryptic pregnancies have been documented across the world for centuries. Historically, when pregnancy diagnoses relied on signs like missed periods and nausea, it was more understandable. Today, with highly accurate modern tests, it is much more straightforward to find out whether you're pregnant, but only if you expect to be pregnant and do a test.

Apparently, there are different reasons why stealth pregnancies can happen and there is no one single factor. However, one of the main causes is hormonal imbalances. This can be because someone has been pregnant and recently given birth, and it takes time to return to normal cycles. The same applies if someone is going through perimenopause and their cycle is not regular. If someone is taking birth control and having unprotected sex, this can lead to a stealth pregnancy, and continuing to take birth control means they might not experience pregnancy symptoms. However, professionals agree that sometimes there does not appear to be an obvious reason for this type of pregnancy.

When Alexis arrived, all close family and friends rallied around and bought her everything she needed, including a cot, bouncy chair, buggy, nappies and babygrows.

'I remember walking into the lounge and thinking, "This is life now." I was so overwhelmed. When we were ready to take her out, we went out and bought our own things, too.'

Kaitlin explains how lucky she felt that her mum was there to support her.

'She was just so calm, which made me feel calmer about it. I think if my mum hadn't been there, the story would be quite different.'

Her husband, Christopher, also sounds like a brilliant support. 'Initially, I think he was quite upset he wasn't there when she was born, but when he came to hospital, he was fully on board with the idea of being a dad. We grew up a lot more after she arrived, but I think because we had been together since we were 13, we were a little bit more mature anyway. It had always been the two of us growing up together.'

Kaitlin explained that she tried to hide it from her friends for as long as she could, but as soon as it came around to her prom, she was meant to be going with her best friend at the time. She didn't have her phone with her, so she couldn't message, and when her dad finally brought her phone to the hospital, there were countless missed calls, wondering where she was.

'I sent her a picture of Alexis, and she replied asking what the hell I was doing babysitting someone's kid when we were going to prom. I then had to tell her she was mine. I quickly FaceTimed her to tell her, and she just sobbed. She had just had her make-up done and it slid down her face! I got her to tell all my classmates because I knew I didn't want to have the conversation over and over again. The teachers at school were told. Generally, everyone was shocked, and I think it probably became more real when my friends visited us when we got home.'

Reflecting on a nurse asking her if she wanted to keep Alexis just after she was born, Kaitlin said that at the time, it 'just went over my head'.

'Thinking back, they were obviously concerned that I might not be able to deal with things, but I have an amazing support network. At the time, I said: "She's mine, and I'm taking her home." '

Kaitlin credits her mum with really helping her find her feet as a mum.

'Having Mum around meant that it all felt quite natural, and every-thing fell into place for us. My mum took the reins and showed me what to do.'

Kaitlin started a new school for sixth form just a few months after Alexis was born.

'I never really had a clear plan of what I wanted to do. I had to stay in education, but I didn't picture going to university. As soon as I had her, I knew it was the right thing to do to stay at school for two years and then find full-time work after that. I had to go in before the term started and tell my teachers what had happened, but they were really good and allowed me to focus on three subjects rather than four.

'Fitting into the schedule of sixth form was quite tricky to start off with. She went to the same nursery that my mum works in as a nursery chef, so that worked out well. If I had an early start, she would just take her with her. She and my dad really helped.'

Kaitlin and Christopher both worked part-time jobs to pay for the nursery costs outside of their funded hours.

'We were able to cover her costs ourselves. We knew that it was something we needed to do and get used to. Me and Chris wanted to do it and pay for things ourselves.'

Teenage motherhood has generally decreased in the past few decades across different parts of the world, including the UK. The under-18 conception rate in England and Wales has decreased significantly since 2007. Between 2007 and 2021, the rate dropped by 68 per cent, from 42 conceptions per 1,000 women to 13 per 1,000 women, resulting in 13,131 under-18 conceptions in 2021.

Kaitlin said she felt slightly 'looked down on' due to her age. 'When I would get on the bus, there would always be comments about how nice it was that I was looking after my niece, and when I told them she was mine, there were always comments about me being too young to have a baby.'

Kaitlin added: 'When I took her to nursery, none of the other mums really spoke to me because I think they naturally steered away from our family. That felt hard. For the same reason, I didn't really go to any of the mum and baby groups because I felt like I would be judged, and there wouldn't be people there who would support us in the way we needed. I found it easier to hang out with my friends and family.

'I just treat her as a gift, and we are like best friends,' she said.

It's a shame, because surely there could be a sense of learning from young mums who have so much to offer. I do think sometimes people have preconceived ideas about what it means to be a young mum and how they have found themselves in that position, but there are pros and cons to doing it earlier or later in life. I grew up with a friend who had her little girl when we were still quite young, and now her daughter has had a daughter, so she is a year older than me, and she is a nan. We never know what will happen in life, and we don't know what is around the corner, but hopefully, she'll have another 50 years with her daughter and granddaughter and get to spend so much of her life with them. What a gift that is. I had Minnie later and crammed a lot into my life before having her. I was 35, turning 36, when I gave birth. In hindsight, I do wish I had started our family a bit earlier.

Kaitlin now works as a bridal consultant in a wedding dress shop. She and Christopher bought their first home and tied the knot in 2023, with Alexis as their flower girl.

'We did it all in the same month.' She laughed. 'Alexis loved our wedding day. Looking back at photos, I can't imagine having a wedding without her being such a big part of our day. It has all worked out for the best.'

When we spoke, Kaitlin also told me she was expecting her second baby – which, she said, she imagines will be an altogether different experience to having Alexis.

'Alexis was a little bit unsure to begin with because she's had us to herself for nine years, but I'm sure she will love getting involved when the baby is here.'

8

'I knew I was one of the lucky ones.'

A story of courage

To my gorgeous girl,

Although you arrived four months early, I knew I was one of the lucky ones. Even after meeting you in the NICU seven hours after giving birth, I knew we were bonded, and I loved you unconditionally whatever was thrown our way, and that was a lot.

I loved you despite your fused eyes, see-through skin, bruised body and tube breathing oxygen into your lungs, and despite not even being technically 'viable' yet.

Pregnancy, for me, just didn't seem to work. I had been sick every day and had been up to the hospital many times with bleeding, but when you were 22+3, my waters broke, and I didn't know what to expect. Sadly for you and me, over the next few days, this led to an infection and sepsis, so you were induced with the expectation that I would cuddle you for the first and last time. I'm so lucky you wouldn't budge, and when we hit 23+0 weeks gestation, you were predicted to be about 500 grams. It opened up the possibility of resuscitating you at birth, and despite the grim statistics and the uncertainty about your future, I couldn't not have a team there to help you in your greatest hour of need.

Before you were born, I asked if you would be a science experiment, as I didn't even know babies could survive this early. Your consultant had reassured me you wouldn't be. But two months later, when you were still ventilated with a collapsed lung and pneumonia whilst withdrawing from morphine from an operation, I really debated what I had done. I hated seeing you in pain. Your tiny body had been through so much, and it was all my fault.

If I had known you would have brain bleeds, two holes in your heart, so many cannulations, blood transfusions and need eye treatment to save your sight, I might have taken a different route. How could you be OK after all of this? How could you fit into this world that had been so cruel to you? For me, it was like watching you drown, but with no water involved. One weekend, your oxygen saturations stayed in the sixties and seventies, yet you were being given 100 per cent oxygen. Each day brought a new challenge.

Whilst other mothers held their baby whenever they liked, it took two or three nurses to get you out of the incubator so your tube didn't dislodge, and then after two hours of cuddling, you were taken off me because you were born during Covid-19 in 2020 and rules dictated I must leave. It broke my heart; it felt so heavy when you were not with me, and I felt such loss; it was all so wrong.

For two months, I could visit you for just two hours a day until, finally, Bliss Charity met with hospitals to work out better visiting hours. I was desperate for you to come home, but your oxygen dependency was still too high even when you finally got off the ventilator.

Five months after you were born, you came home, tube-fed and still on oxygen that would continue for a year and a half. Getting you home was the best day of my life. I still didn't

Dear Minnie

know if you would be 'OK', whatever that meant, but as long as we were together, I knew we would cope. I was fine that the house looked like a hospital, and at first, I kept you on monitors day and night to make sure you were still getting enough oxygen. Having you in your cot next to me was what I'd been waiting for, and my heart could start healing after all our time separated. I could eat again and smile and plan a future despite being exhausted with your monitors waking me up 15–20 times a night. Finally, your nana and auntie could meet you. At five months old and 8lb you were home.

I wish back then I could have told myself that, three years later, you would be able to walk and run and put words together to ask me for a snack every five minutes and enjoy Peppa Pig like other children your age. What relief I would have felt to know you would be a happy three-year-old who's not in pain and has a life ahead of her. Although speech can still be challenging for you, and you are held back more than your peers with appointments and check-ups, which you have to miss nursery for, these appointments are becoming less and less as the years go by.

I will tell you about all the other premature babies before you, the ones that didn't go home, including two of your friends from the hospital. How the trial and error, science and determination from dedicated doctors, nurses and researchers over many years meant that in 2020, a baby at 23 weeks and 0 days did have a chance, despite the difficult journey it involved.

With your birth, the worst nightmare that could have happened began before turning into the most wonderful dream I could have imagined, and for someone born so small, your strength and determination astound me.

Love Mum

***

Wʜᴇɴ ɪ ᴛᴀʟᴋᴇᴅ ᴛᴏ ᴛʜɪs lovely mum, Emma, about her experience of being in hospital with her premature baby during the Covid-19 pandemic, she admitted that she is still not emotionally recovered from having to leave her baby but is so grateful her daughter is now at home and thriving.

'I remember every day how lucky I have been. She has beaten so many odds,' she said. 'We spoke to one of her paediatric doctors recently, and he talked about her being one of his big success stories,' she said. 'I feel lucky after the experiences I have seen in NICU.'

A preterm delivery occurs when a baby is born before completing 37 weeks of gestation (37 weeks being considered full term). Across the world, over 10 per cent of pregnancies result in preterm births. Extreme prematurity is before 28 weeks. Once a baby reaches 23 to 24 weeks, they have a chance of survival outside of the womb with intensive medical treatment. The NHS states that even with intensive treatment, five out of ten babies born at this gestation will not make it. One out of ten will have a serious disability, and four will not have a serious disability but may have health problems and challenges in childhood.

Research indicates that more babies born at 22 weeks are now surviving and being discharged from the hospital due to recent changes in national guidelines. Previously, until 2019, UK hospitals only provided treatment to save the lives of babies born at 23 weeks or later. However, new guidelines from the British Association of Perinatal Medicine, introduced in October of that year, reflect advancements in neonatal and obstetric care that have improved survival rates for extremely premature infants. The updated guidelines now recommend offering 'survival-focused care', such as respiratory support, to babies born at 22 weeks' gestation. This care should be provided following a risk assessment and in consultation with the parents. Although overall survival rates for babies born at 22 weeks remain low, a study has found that a greater number of these infants are now surviving to be discharged from the hospital and receiving treatment compared to before. The research involved 1,001 babies who were alive at the start of labour at 22 weeks' gestation.

These premature babies are affectionately called 'preemies' on maternity units. Before I was a mum, I made a film in lockdown in a Bradford hospital about premature babies for BBC's *Panorama*, and they were just so tiny. I was so starry-eyed around the doctors. I could not believe the work they did when the babies were so, so small. Babies born this early can sometimes weigh the same as a small bag of sugar. The NICU is the most humbling space, with parents sitting by their babies' incubators and doctors who are the best of humanity. I was so in awe of them. It feels like a very special and nurturing place. Seeing this amazing work and sitting alongside new parents as their baby received crucial specialist help gave me a new appreciation for the NHS. Looking at the wall of thank you cards, the care they give to so, so many families and the lives they have saved feel always unquantifiable.

Emma explained that her situation was tough because she could not stay with her baby in the hospital due to the Covid-19 rules at the time, so she was forced to come and go during the allocated visiting hours.

'There were some days when she had to be torn out of my arms because visiting hours were over,' she explained. 'I trusted the nurses with her life, yet they were the ones who had to take her from me. Sometimes, she would stop breathing, and she would be being resuscitated at the same time that it was my time to leave. They would breathe for her with a neo-puff. I never saw chest compressions, but they were bringing her back, and I was being told I could not stay there. I could still cry about that now because it makes me angry.'

Unlike many parents who are nervous about returning home with their baby after an extended stay in the NICU, Emma could not wait for her daughter to leave the hospital.

'I was so happy to leave,' she said softly. 'I know other people say they feel quite safe in the NICU and are worried about taking their child home, but I wanted to get back home.'

Emma's daughter was on oxygen at home for a year and a half. 'I had a SATs monitor on her, and it would beep every time she shook her leg in her sleep, and I would wake up. I couldn't not have it on because I was so worried she'd stop breathing. She has chronic lung disease. But you wouldn't know it, and we are hopeful she will grow out of it.'

We spoke of the extraordinary pressure these parents are under. Emma told us that after a year, she still felt that she couldn't return to work as a member of cabin crew on an airline. She called to tell her boss, and they agreed she could have a year of unpaid leave.

'I was off work until she was two, so I feel happy I got to keep my job. I thought I would have to be a stay-at-home mum. Luckily, I am just part-time now. I have only left her for two nights, but I feel differently about work now that I'm a mum.'

When people ask how old her daughter is, Emma explains that because she is so small, she normally tells them why.

'Some people will ask how early she was and say, "Oh, I know a 36-weeker!" I know it's all valid, as the babies they know are still premature, but I wish I had gotten that far.'

Emma talked about the support she has from her mum and sister. Her daughter is at a nursery they both like and has an EHCP (an education, health and care plan), so she will get extra help.

'But this is a lot less than we thought she might need,' she explained. 'Just the fact she can communicate with me is amazing.'

She also spoke of the fact that her daughter is catching up with her peers. Even though she has been put back a year, so she will have an extra year at nursery before starting school, Emma is having similar challenges to other parents.

'When she was little, I couldn't relate to other parents because the issues they were facing were so different to my issues, but now I definitely can more. Now I think we can chat about the same things. I'm back on "normal parenting" mode. Stuff like not wanting to clean her teeth.

'She's fine – I'm not worried about milestones or anything like that. I didn't even think we would reach them. I don't know how we got away with it, but I'm so thankful that we did.'

9

'I am the mum you deserve to have.'

A story of growth

Dear Evie,

When I became pregnant with you, I felt scared and confused, but also an overwhelming sense of love and the need to protect you.

You already had three much older siblings who lived with your Nannie and then your auntie because I had spent 15 years addicted to heroin and crack cocaine and had been to prison on numerous occasions for shoplifting to fund my addiction. I definitely wasn't the mum to them that they deserved to have or needed me to be, or the mum that I wished I had been.

When you were conceived, I had already been drug-free for six months, so when I discovered that I was pregnant with you, I knew that I wanted things to be different and to be the mum that you needed me to be. It was during my last prison sentence in 2018 that I made the decision that I wasn't going to use drugs when I got out of prison. Your sister Ebonie wouldn't let me be a part of my granddaughter Elodie's life because she didn't want me in and out of her life as I had been with her. I had already detoxed while in prison, which was really hard, but somehow, I found the will-power to not use when I got out and attended day programmes and surrounded myself with people who weren't taking drugs. It was difficult, but I did it and didn't go back to using drugs and started seeing my family more.

Your biological father was very abusive, violent and controlling towards me. He regu-larly attacked me, so when I was five months pregnant, I moved 200 miles away into a women's refuge where I got support and the help I needed to not return to the violent relationship I had with your biological father. While at the refuge, I had key work sessions and made friendships with other women who were in the same situation. I began to plan for your arrival. I lived near the seaside, so I would go for walks with the other women on the beach and began to realise what a 'normal life' could be. I was able to think for myself and make my own decisions, and I started to feel more independent, which I loved.

When you were born, social services came to the hospital to say that they were taking me to court to try and have you removed from my care because they were concerned I would go back to the violent relationship or could end up relapsing. I have never been so scared in my whole life, as losing you was not an option. The love I felt for you was more than I can explain. You were, and still are, so perfect. The thought of having you removed from my care was the scariest thing I've ever experienced. I couldn't sleep as I didn't want to miss a minute with you; I just wanted to hold you and never let you go. I genuinely felt that I wouldn't be able to live if you were taken away from me. I was so worried and knew that your older sister and brothers would never forgive me if you were taken away, so I felt like I would have been losing all four of my children.

Luckily the courts didn't agree with social services and didn't feel that there were enough grounds to remove my tiny baby from my care, but instead, it was agreed that I would go to Trevi House in Plymouth. Trevi House is a mother-and-baby rehab where we spent the first eight months of our life together. While I was there, I did a lot of work on myself around domestic abuse, addiction and past traumas. I received counselling, key work sessions and group therapy. I did everything asked of me and felt very determined to get it right and be a good mum.

I loved you so much. Waking up to your smiling face and watching you grow was the best feeling. I loved taking you to soft play, singing songs and nursery rhymes with you, reading you stories and giving you lots of cuddles. There was no way I was going to lose you, so am so grateful that I got the opportunity to go to Trevi and get all the help, support and therapy that I got there.

In the mornings, I would get you up, get us both ready for the day, and you would go into the on-site nursery while I attended groups, then I would pick you up at lunchtime and spend time with you until afternoon sessions started, when I would take you back to the nursery. We would spend our evenings and spare time in the communal area with the other mums and children. We would go on outings at weekends to the beach, parks and aquarium, which you loved. I made some good friends, some of whom I still have contact with now. We all supported each other and became like a little community. I learnt to deal with traumas and be the best version of myself. I am the mum that you deserve to have.

After eight months, we left Trevi and moved into our own little flat. Leaving Trevi was quite emotional, but I was so excited to be starting the next chapter of our life and so determined to continue on the right track and give you a childhood that you will look back on with love and happiness.

You are now five years old and have your own challenges due to autism and being non-verbal, but you are surrounded by love and encouragement. I now know what a healthy relationship looks like, thanks to the relationship I have with your stepdad.

You now have a younger sister, Elsie, who you love and who is like your little best friend. You love to play with dollies, dress up, go to the park together and watch a Disney film together. Elsie always follows you around and sees you as her hero, and I have worked hard to rebuild my relationships with your older sister and brothers.

I now have a life that I am proud of. I do a lot of volunteering to help support other women who are experiencing similar things to what I have managed to survive and am now living the life that I was always meant to live. Most importantly, I am a good mum to all five of my children.

I will always love and protect you, advocate for you, and will be your voice until you find your own.

Lots of love, kisses and hugs,

Love Mummy xxx

***

I WAS REALLY KEEN TO include a story from the women's charity Trevi, which runs a residential rehabilitation centre for mothers and their children. It provides a space for women to recover and heal from trauma or domestic violence. They offer therapeutic support in the community and parenting support. I recorded a podcast about making fresh starts and was blown away by the women there and the work they do, and there was one woman in particular who had been struggling with addiction for years and years. She lived in London, not far from where I was living at the time, and she was so smitten with her little girl, who was dressed immaculately. It wasn't planned that I would speak to her, but I bumped into her in the centre, and we got chatting. I wasn't a mum when I spoke to her and now I realise that trying to navigate your way through motherhood is hard enough, and there were so many extra things she was battling. I really felt like I wanted to speak to someone who had successfully turned their life around and I was grateful for Tammy telling me her remarkable story of growth, which is beautifully intertwined with the birth of her daughter Evie.

She spoke about her life, spending years being in and out of prison and not really feeling like she was a mum to her older kids.

'Even when I did see them, I wasn't consistent. Sometimes, I would have to cut it short as I was starting to get withdrawal symptoms and needed to go and get more drugs. It was awful.'

The last time Tammy went to prison, she was sent to an open prison in Kent, and it was looking at a picture of her granddaughter that she had taken off the internet that spurred her on to make a change. Considering the challenges she faced back then, she spoke incredibly eloquently about how she recognised that she wanted something different to the path she had gone down.

'I looked at this photo, and I knew I had to be in that little girl's life,' she told me. 'I had tried changing for my children in the past, but I wasn't ready. Not because I didn't love them enough or they weren't important enough, but because my daughter did not want me to be a part of her daughter's life. She didn't want me in and out of her life, like I had been with her. She wouldn't let me see her, and I only had the pictures because I had got them off Facebook. The next time I got out, I never used [drugs] again.'

Tammy now has four grandchildren, but she describes the eldest as 'the little girl who saved my life'.

'If it weren't for her, I would probably be dead,' she explained. 'My sister used to think she would have to sit down with my eldest children and tell them that I had been found dead in a ditch from an overdose or something like that. Luckily, I managed to turn it around.'

Tammy also spoke about a conversation she had with a prison officer during her last stint inside.

'They sent me to an open prison, even though I didn't meet the criteria. Once I was there, they didn't know what to do with me, but I stayed. One day, I asked a prison officer why I was there as no one wanted to give me an opportunity to change. He said to me, "Believe in yourself, because I believe in you."

'Those words stuck with me forever because no one had ever said they believed in me before. I don't think he probably did believe in me – he didn't really know enough about me. But it made a huge difference to my life'.

There are many women in prison. The Prison Reform Trust estimates that around 17,000 children are impacted by maternal imprisonment each year. For the children who are living with their mothers, 95 per cent of them have to leave their homes because their mother going to prison means they will have no one to look after them. I filmed with a couple of mums in prison in America, and we shot this heartbreaking scene where one of the mum's two kids, who were in foster care, came into the prison to visit. What really stayed with me was how familiar the kids were with the prison. They knew they had to put their hands up and opened their mouths when they were walking through security. The prison officers didn't tell them what to do; they did it automatically. It was clearly something they had been used to since they were tiny. It felt so bleak.

Tammy started rebuilding her relationship with her older children, spending a Christmas together, which she hadn't done for years. After she had been out of prison for six months, she found out she was pregnant. She had been in an abusive relationship for around five years. She moved to a refuge to escape her partner, but when her daughter was born, social services told her that Trevi was her last chance to keep her baby.

'When I was in the hospital, and I was given paperwork to go to court so my baby would be taken away, I remember being so scared of losing her. If I had lost Evie, I would've lost my other children because they never would've forgiven me for that. I knew that if they took my child, I would go and find the nearest drug dealer and take an overdose. I couldn't have lived my life like that. It would've been a very selfish thing to do, but that is how messed up my head was at the time.

'I knew I needed to do whatever it took, and it was the best thing that could ever have happened to me. I cannot shout Trevi's praises enough. I had to put in the hard work, but they gave me the tools I needed. I couldn't have done it without them. It has changed my life, and it is sad that more women don't get the same help.'

Tammy now has another child with her new partner and is reconciled with her older children. She was babysitting one of her older son's babies the day we spoke – a little girl.

'The fact he trusts me to have her means a lot,' she said, while carefully adjusting her baby granddaughter's headband.

She also plans to be honest with her younger daughters about her experience.

'I don't think there is anything to gain from not being honest with them,' she said in a matter-of-fact tone. 'Hopefully, if I tell them about my experience with drugs, they will see how much it messed up my life and will not go near them.'

Tammy now runs outreach support for Trevi. Her personal experience means that she is perfectly placed to help other people going through similar challenges.

'I love the work that I do, and I can relate to the women I work with. They know my story,' she told me. 'If I can give one person a tiny bit of hope so they know that it can be done, then everything I have gone through in my life makes it worth it. Once upon a time, I thought I would be an addict forever who couldn't be saved. But I have done it.'

10

'So off I went to throw my best moves on the dance floor.'

A story of unexpected labour

Dear Annabelle,

I was 33 weeks pregnant with you, and it was my cousin's wedding in Cyprus. You were my first baby, and I was more than ready for your arrival as the hyperemesis had become unbearable. Unfortunately, your dad didn't come with us as he was unable to take leave from work.

I had planned to go to the wedding as soon as I got the invite, but the first date had been cancelled due to Covid-19, and at this point, I wasn't even with your dad, never mind pregnant. I was over the moon to be there in the sunshine, ready to celebrate their happy ever after.

Your Granpie (grandad) had begged me not to go to the wedding, as he feared I'd go into labour. But Mummy, knowing best, ignored him, and we went off to the wedding, with the doctors' sign-off.

The night before the wedding, all the guests went on a party boat aptly named the Wave Dancer. *So, of course, I had to be the first on the dance floor to experience dancing with the waves. Whilst doing the awkward shuffle to the dance floor – POP – I felt a strange sensation and became drenched; I looked at my cousin Allan, whose leg was wet, and looked at my dress – and just like in the movies when someone's waters break, I was soaked.*

I paused for a second, everything went into slow motion, and then off I ran to the toilet, followed by all the female members of the family and the captain of the party boat, who came to have a nosey whilst my knickers were around my ankles. Auntie Susan, a retired midwife, then sniffed the liquid and proceeded to tell me I'd wet myself due to my overenthusiastic dancing, so of course, I had to pull myself together and get on with the partying.

So off I went to throw my best moves on the dance floor whilst having mild contractions . . . splits, twerk, splits, funky chicken . . . I was rocking the floor whilst telling everyone I'd just wet myself.

In all honesty, I was so embarrassed that I'd caused a big scene the day before the wedding, potentially ruined the wedding, and all the attention was on me. All whilst my cousin was begging me to give birth in the middle of the aisle the next day. Everyone else thought it was hilarious that I'd 'wet myself'. However, I knew I was in labour but knew nobody else could know, and for that to happen, I had to believe it was just wee.

The next day, I went to the wedding and continued to party like nothing was wrong. The stronger the contractions and the more fluid left my body, the more nervous I felt. But at this point, I didn't dare spoil the wedding.

Dear Minnie

The day after the wedding, I knew I was going to have to go to hospital, so I had to come clean to your grandma and tell her we needed to go and see a medical professional. At this point, I had to ring your dad whilst he was playing cricket and tell him that I was potentially in labour and that he may have to come to Cyprus. However, he wouldn't actually be able to join me whilst I gave birth. He just laughed the phone call off and continued to play cricket, ignoring any further phone calls. I don't think he believed me as a couple of days had gone by since the 'wetting myself' incident, so he thought if I were in labour, I'd have surely given birth by now! Also, he knows I'm a drama queen.

The hospital swabs and scans confirmed that my waters had gone and that I was in labour. The consultant shouted at your grandma for not taking me to hospital sooner as there was not enough amniotic fluid, so she felt guilty but had no idea I was in labour. Due to the language barrier, she just sat there stunned and worrying. The doctors carried on doing tests on me without telling me what was going on, and all of a sudden, my bladder felt empty; I just remember turning to your grandma and exclaiming, 'I've just had a magic wee,' not realising I'd been catheterised, so we had a good belly laugh about this, which did help settle our nerves. Unfortunately, due to the Covid-19 restrictions in the hospital, this was the last time anyone could join me in the hospital, which was so worrying for me, especially as I wasn't offered a translator.

A day later, the contractions got stronger, and I was praying for you to have a Cypriot passport! I was dreaming about moving over there if you got dual citizenship. However, the hospital managed to stop the labour with medication. After a three-night stay in the hospital, I had to catch an early flight home by myself as there was only one seat left on the plane. I was absolutely petrified I would give birth in the air and that it wouldn't be safe, but I knew we were better at home with your daddy. During the flight, I just remember concentrating on my breathing and rehearsing what I was going to say to the air stewards if I did start having contractions again: 'Excuse me, have you ever laboured a baby before?' Or should I just jump up and say, 'Is there a midwife on this plane?'

No doctors could give us the 'OK' to fly, but they indicated that if I somehow did get home, it would be ideal. Your grandad dropped us at the airport before he went out for cocktails for tea with grandma and Auntie Amelia to calm their nerves! After the most nerve-wracking four-hour flight home, we landed in the early hours in Manchester to be greeted by your daddy.

When we got home, I had a couple of hours of sleep, and then we went to the hospital, where they kept a close eye on us for the next few weeks.

As the weeks went by, your movements reduced, and my blood pressure went sky-high, which I can only assume was due to sheer panic, so I was induced. Whilst in labour, your heart rate dropped, so I had to have an episiotomy, and you were suctioned out.

As I didn't know your gender, the midwife passed you to me, and I was screaming for someone to 'take this baby off me', as I thought the worst had happened. The crash team ran in to resuscitate you, as you needed help with your breathing, and to take you down to NICU, where you spent your next few days until you were ready to come home.

Those few weeks were the most exciting and craziest of my life, but they were worth it for you.

Dear Minnie

Of course, your first holiday abroad last year was to Cyprus! I can't wait until we are there again with the whole family doing the funky chicken and hopefully not wetting ourselves!!

Lots of love,

Mummy

***

I REALLY WANTED TO INCLUDE an unexpected birth story, as I think many births don't necessarily go according to plan.

'It's such a random story,' Lizzie concedes, chuckling and hugging her younger daughter Xanthe, who when we spoke was four months old and snoozing in her arms. 'Everyone I tell asks me: "Why were you on a party boat?!" I was on the boat, and everything was fine. We had eaten – there were 20 of us up this long table – and the music came on. One person gave me the nod to get up and dance. I am the idiot who will always get up and dance, and all of a sudden, there was water everywhere. It was all up one of my relative's legs. Then I ran, followed by 15 people, into this cubicle, with the captain following all of us. I think I knew deep down it was my waters, but I felt like if a midwife was telling me it was just wee, maybe it was just wee. I was having mild contractions all through the wedding but then got on to the dance floor that night again and did the splits and more twerking.'

Lizzie, who is blonde and athletic, explained her willingness to show off her dancing skills.

'I used to be a pole-dancing instructor, and my aunty said: "If she is doing those moves, it's 100 per cent not her waters."'

Eventually, when she got checked out at a local centre and the doctors confirmed it was her waters, Lizzie said she felt petrified.

'First, we were going to try to get my partner to fly out with a car seat just in case. Once the labour had stopped, I knew I could go home. My mum was going to come with me, but only one seat was left on the plane.'

However, the situation became even more stressful when she was asked to get off.

'You know what it's like when some airlines oversell the tickets. They were asking people to not get on the flight. They said they would ask people to volunteer not to get the flight, but if no one did, they would start randomly picking people. I was worried I was going to be booted off. In the end, luckily, I was fine.

'It was so scary flying by myself. I had felt minor contractions, but I wondered how you are supposed to know when you are going to give birth. By that point, they had fully stopped, and I got back OK.'

It is normal to have contractions a few weeks before giving birth. These are called Braxton Hicks. Some doctors and midwives believe that they contribute to toning the uterine muscles and enhancing blood flow to the placenta.

Lizzie's birth – a few weeks after her return to the UK – was very stressful due to the fact her baby needed time in NICU.

'There was silence in the room immediately after and that wasn't how I imagined it would be. She was taken away, and it was a few days before any of us got to hold her. It was so scary. Obviously, she is absolutely fine now and people have it a lot worse. But in those first moments and days, it wasn't how I imagined it was going to be.'

When I asked her if she stayed at home during her second pregnancy, Lizzie told me she had been persuaded abroad again.

'Everyone wanted to go on holiday. I didn't want to go, but it was six weeks earlier in my pregnancy than it had been the time before.' She laughed. 'You would've really thought that I had learnt my lesson the first time, but I went – and everything was fine.'

11

'Watching you grow is the most wonderful gift.'

A story of discovery

To Millie,

What a journey we have had together so far. It's been four years of adventuring, experiencing and learning together. I wanted to tell you a little bit about when we first met.

Before you read more, I want to explain that you'll read about how sometimes I was sad. There were some things that I didn't understand, and sometimes, when you don't understand, it can make you worry, and that can make you sad. Most importantly, I want you to know that I'm not sad anymore.

Let's go back to the beginning . . .

Your dad and I had travelled from London, where we lived at the time, to Norfolk for a holiday to prepare for your arrival. Or so we thought. It was while we were away that you decided you wanted to join us, too. Seven weeks early, just 1 hour 20 minutes of labour, miles from home and no baby clothes, pushchairs or even a crib purchased. Here you were, our dream baby girl that we had been so excited about meeting.

I can still remember lying in the hospital bed the night you were born. You had been taken off to the special baby care unit to make sure you could breathe OK, which you were brilliant at and didn't need any help with. But you needed help with feeding, as those skills hadn't developed yet. Your dad had given you your first bit of milk earlier and then headed back to our holiday home. We only had a small cuddle before you were taken away. It all felt so surreal and like nothing had happened. I don't think I slept for a minute.

The morning came and it was time to visit you. You were tiny. Lying there, swaddled in a blanket in an open incubator. You had a tube into your nose, which was how you were fed, but otherwise, you looked so peaceful. There she is, my daughter, I thought.

'She doesn't look how I imagined,' I remember saying to your dad. I couldn't quite put my finger on it. Your eyes didn't look like mine; they were more oval, and your face looked round. But I didn't think any more of it. I was still in shock; I hadn't really slept, and we hadn't met before. How would I know how you were going to look?

The nurses helped us get you out of your incubator for our first proper cuddles. As I held you close to my skin, a glow flowed through me, and it all started to sink in – the adrenaline was wearing off, and everything felt calm. The doctors and nurses said how well you were doing. Then we found out something special about you.

'Perhaps we could go into the side room?' the consultant said. I immediately felt a knot in my stomach. As we entered the room, the adrenaline came back. A windowless room, with some chairs and a box of tissues. Why are we here? I thought. Everyone has said how well you're doing. I've seen it myself.

The consultant was a kind, gentle man. 'Your daughter has signs of trisomy 21. Down syndrome,' he said. 'There's nothing to be sorry about. I'm not going to say "sorry". She's going to live a full life just like any other child.'

Dear Minnie

Both your dad and I were shocked, scared and confused. I didn't understand what this meant for us. And I didn't understand how it could have happened. We had the prenatal tests. And whilst I had felt sick most of my pregnancy, everything had been straightforward.

Then, so many thoughts and questions ran through my mind: am I going to have to give up everything to care for you? What will your future look like? Will you know you have Down syndrome? Will we ever connect as a mother and daughter? How will I protect you from a world that can sometimes be so harsh, judgemental and not inclusive? What will happen when your dad and I aren't here? This is different; how do I do different?

The next few days and weeks were like a blur. We did a lot of research, and some days, I just wanted to forget about Down syndrome. I didn't want to talk about it. I just wanted to think about you as Millie, as a baby, just like any other.

Like every new parent, it was time for the Instagram announcement. We had to tell everyone about the arrival of our beautiful girl, but we also had to tell them that you had Down syndrome. I remember feeling nervous. Were people going to judge me? What were people going to say? But I needn't have been. The support was amazing. People who I hadn't spoken to for years were suddenly there. Sharing their love and compassion. But most importantly, just talking to me like any other mum of a newborn baby.

We went back to London, and you stayed in the hospital for four weeks. I would sit by your bedside for 13 hours every day. Cuddling, feeding you, watching you sleep (you slept a lot).

Leaving you every day was the hardest thing, and when I wasn't with you, I felt sad. Sad that you weren't there with me. That the start of our life together wasn't how I'd imagined. And I was sad that you had Down syndrome. You were the most beautiful person I had ever seen. And now Down syndrome was going to take that all away, I thought. From you, and me.

Once you were home, I don't think I stopped cuddling you. I carried you everywhere in my carrier. Holding you close, walking proudly through the streets. My beautiful baby. We could finally be together and bond. The fog was starting to clear and I was starting to see that everything was going to be OK. Yes, our journey was going to be a little different, but I started to understand that the difference wasn't bad. It was just that, different. And what I had importantly learnt from all of this was that so many journeys are.

And now you're four. Watching you grow is the most wonderful gift. You are kind, funny, smart and cheeky. You love to sing, dance and play babies, and hide and seek. And our bond is so strong.

When you learn something new, my heart fills with joy. One of my biggest joys has been to see you walk and run around. You found it hard to walk, always preferring a bottom shuffle, then one day, on Father's Day, a couple of months before your fourth birthday, you just stood up and walked across the room. Your face lit up and you gave yourself a little clap at the end. Then you just stood up and did it again and again and again. I couldn't have felt prouder of you, and I was so excited to see your happiness in having mastered it. Yes, it can feel frustrating sometimes that some of the skills take a little longer to master, but then once you do, the excitement of seeing you do something that I often take for granted as being so simple makes it all worth it. We don't take anything for granted and celebrate every success, no matter how small. And I wouldn't ever change those feelings.

But you also bring so much joy to others. All those worries about judgement, and our experience so far has been so positive. At a toddler event, another parent once said,

'She just lights up the room,' and I see this being the effect you bring to so many places we go and people we see. You go to a mainstream nursery where you are really popular. When you left your last preschool, your key worker shed a little tear on your last day.

'Thank you for letting us be part of her journey,' she said.

You bring something to people's lives that you can't just get everywhere.

Soon, it will be time for school, and I can't wait to experience this next chapter with you. To help and support you through this next phase of learning and watch as you grow into a young girl.

Love Mummy

***

WHEN I SPOKE WITH LOUISE, we talked about the doctor who delivered the news about Millie's diagnosis.

'He was very kind and approached it in just the right way. I know some parents have had experiences of nurses crying or everyone telling them they are sorry. That is not right.'

Down syndrome is a condition in which a person has an extra chromosome. The negativity and stereotypes surrounding having a baby with Down syndrome often arise from a mix of societal attitudes, misconceptions rooted in past understanding, and fear of the unknown. In the past, there was a belief that children with Down syndrome had very limited potential in terms of learning, development and independence. It was believed that they could not achieve meaningful milestones or lead fulfilling lives.

Now, more is understood about the condition; children with Down syndrome will experience some level of learning disability, but most will learn to read and write and may attend mainstream schools. They should be given the same opportunities as any other child. Although there are several health conditions associated with Down syndrome, with proper treatment and medical care, children can overcome these challenges and thrive.

When I asked her what she initially thought her life would be like as a mother of a baby with Down syndrome, she answered thoughtfully: 'At first, I had a flash of all sorts of thoughts. Initially, you have no idea, and then your brain tries to start filling in the gaps. Thoughts came, like – "I am going to have to be a carer and quit everything." One of the strongest feelings I have heard from the community is the thought that you will never go on holiday again. I guess that's a reflection of feeling like you might not have an independent family unit. You feel like you have this picture of parenthood and family life, and then you are given the news that your child is different, and it's like the piece of paper becomes blank again.'

She continued: 'Other than googling a lot of stuff, I followed other families on Instagram. I joined a Down Syndrome UK online group and a therapy group that was based near where I was living then in London.

'When you become a mother, you need to find your identity again. Layered on top of that, with Millie having Down syndrome – you enter this community, and I started to see lots of people who go down the advocacy route, where it is all about projecting a positive message of getting out there and sharing that message. Then there were mums learning the sign language, Makaton, and having "wine and sign" nights. I entered some of these groups, but within them, I was trying to find my place. I didn't really know where I wanted to sit.

'I remember going to a speech and language group and was quite nervous. I remember walking in and looking around the room and thinking, "Oh, these people look like me." I was surprised that other people, like me, have children with Down syndrome. I felt a real feeling of relief. I have always sat on the edge of these groups but have been grateful for them.'

The issue of language is one Louise rightly feels passionately about. 'Sometimes there is this tendency to refer to people with Down syndrome as "they", such as "they are so joyful" or whatever it may be, as if they all share the same or similar characteristics. Millie is actually quite reserved, and children or people with Down syndrome are obviously all different people. I remember once I was in a shop, and a woman made a reference to "she's not totally Down's", and I kept trying to correct her and tell her that it was not something you could have a bit of. In the end, it felt like a lost cause and like I just needed to get out of there.'

She has also noticed this with medical professionals. Some people with Down syndrome have heart-related conditions, and once, when they were at the hospital, there was an assumption that Millie did, too.

I made a documentary for my TV series with a family whose son, Lucas, had Down syndrome. I found it really insightful, and that family echoed much of what Louise was saying. We have an idea of what Down syndrome can look like and what it means, but every child is different. The little boy in the documentary was an absolute delight and an example of Down syndrome not being his entire identity. I remember talking to Lucas's mum about the language that people use around Down syndrome and how they had to learn how to educate an older family member about the right way to speak about their son's condition.

Louise says she feels that, as parents, we are all triggered by different things and for her, it is the trisomy or Down syndrome test, which is done when the fetus is between 10 and 14 weeks old to assess the chances of your baby having Down syndrome, Edwards' syndrome or Patau's syndrome. It is called a combined test because it involves both an ultrasound scan and a blood test. The blood test can be performed simultaneously with the 12-week scan. If you opt for the test, a blood sample will be collected. During the scan, the fluid at the back of the baby's neck, known as 'nuchal translucency', will be measured. Your age and the results from these two tests are then used to calculate the likelihood of the baby having Down syndrome, Edwards' syndrome or Patau's syndrome. This screening is optional, and if you decide to go ahead with it and are found to have a high chance of having a baby with one of these conditions, you can choose to have further tests.

'The idea is that this test is to see whether your baby has a high chance of having Down syndrome. A test to see if your baby is like mine. And often then a consideration from the parents on whether they wish to proceed with the pregnancy. I understand why someone might make that decision because they do not know what it means to be a parent with a child with Down syndrome, and they are understandably fearful. Of course, this isn't always the choice that people make. But I feel it in my chest when someone talks to me or asks me about it. "But didn't you have the test?" some people would say.'

What has surprised Louise the most about being Millie's mum? 'I am constantly surprised by how capable she is and how kind and open people are. Some things can be harder, and there's some extra parenting to do for sure, but there's lots of similarities in terms of the struggles and the joys that any parent goes through with a toddler or bringing up a child. It's just different, and what motherhood, and perhaps particularly being the mother of a child who has a disability, has shown me is that everyone's experiences are different.'

12

'No matter the journey, we are perfect for each other.'

A story of adoption

To our girls,

Not many parents can honestly say that they brought their second baby home for the first time on the way back from Disneyland, but we did just that. We are conditioned to believe that parenthood through adoption will be a long process and that whirlwind deliveries only take place during mad dashes to the hospital, but in very different circumstances, the two of you managed to take us by surprise in the most unexpected of ways. We became first-time parents on nine days' notice and our second adoption took less than three months from start to finish. Your journey to us is one for the ages.

Our experience of adoption was hard and fast; once the decision to adopt was made, we threw ourselves into the unknown, believing that the only way forward was to do everything a social worker said or our chances of becoming parents would be snatched away. Six months of free therapy with our beautifully blunt social worker began. We were forced to confront memories, childhood trauma and our darkest secrets whilst simultaneously holding it together, so as not to seem too damaged by anything we discussed. *Vivid memories: quitting smoking to 'get an under-five-year-old' (notwithstanding one blip in a north London pub when I convinced myself that a social worker had seen me and parenthood was lost forever), losing three stone (via a 600-calorie-a-day diet) for fear of not passing a medical, being picked up off the kitchen floor by our best friend because the pressure was just too much. But then, from nowhere, it happened. Who knew you could fall in love with a photograph?*

One hundred and twenty families wanted you, our tiny little Bean, and you were going to be ours. The day we met you was a blur of love and confusion. You smiled instantly, giant brown eyes and the most perfect skin. I wanted to take you and run, but we had two weeks of transition to wait. No one prepared me for the alien feeling of falling instantly in love with my baby and then being forced to walk away day after day, watching another woman bathe you in a way that I never would, asking for permission to hold you, my daughter, and becoming disproportionately angry at the lurid pink babygrows covered in diamante and frills that made you, my child, look like someone else's dress-up game. I remember endless hours sitting in roadworks around the North Circular following long days packing up at work, and maternity leave starting after just a few days' notice. Two hours from Wood Green to Hanger Lane and back again, day after day. I still can't listen to Adele's 21 without vivid flashbacks to this time.

At home, our family and friends spent days clearing and decorating your bedroom like an episode of Changing Rooms, *just in time for Christmas. The decision had been ours: to finish work and be ready for our first child within nine days, or wait three months and have you bounce between foster placements before finally coming to us. I've never seen a Mamas and Papas salesperson smile so broadly as when we walked through the door and said, 'We need everything for a baby, but we need it to take away today, please.'*

The caveats, though – 'Take down your Christmas decorations or she'll attach the trauma of change to the fairy lights; make sure her bedroom's ready, there'll be too much difference otherwise; send toys to get used to; don't forget to sleep with a scarf in your bed so she recognises your smell.' You were six months old. There are so many ways in which we felt we could break this and get it wrong for you within the blink of an eye. So when that magical homecoming day finally came, what did we do on the way home? We stopped off at Brent Cross for a poke about the shops, of course.

The haze of confusion of those early days was mind-blowing. You had a raging chest infection and chronic reflux and were so, so tiny. You were six months old, wearing four-month-old clothes; I rocked you on our first night together as your nose bled, Mama panicked and I cried. I wanted my mum, but she wasn't allowed to come. 'Create a bubble', 'prioritise the new bond', the social worker said – after six months of 'proving the strength of our support network', we weren't allowed to call upon them in our first days of parenthood.

The weeks passed, and the world kept turning. As our world opened up, we watched everyone who met you fall for you as quickly as we had. These were my happiest days; proudly walking you across Alexandra Palace Park through the rain to playgroup, watching your eyes open up to the magic of the world around you, the happiest, most charming little lady I had ever met. I literally couldn't love you more.

Then the phone call came. 'There's a challenge to the adoption – but don't worry, they're almost never successful.' On a KIT (keeping in touch) day at work, I collapsed to the floor. It was the first time I'd ever had a panic attack. There were three further months of waiting for our final court date, the bit that no one knows about until they've been through it. You have to wait for the adoption order. This meant at least six months of possible challenge when you could have been snatched away in an instant. I remember crying in Nana and Grandad's hallway, making plans for how we'd run away to family abroad; how if you were taken away from me, every piece of you needed to be taken from our home without me having to see. I watched my own mum's face crumble in helplessness. I had to be strong for you, but in that moment, I was about as far from OK as any parent could possibly be. We had no control over what would happen – you were the centre of our world, and even the smallest risk of you being taken from us was impossible to tolerate. Then, from nowhere, it was done. Your surname was changed, adoption order granted, and life could begin again.

As the years passed, we moved away from London to the seaside. There was a beach at the end of the road, and our family was around the corner. Life felt perfectly still. You were thriving and so settled but also desperate for a sibling. Our perfect girl, we couldn't believe that lightning would strike twice. Surely, we'd never be so lucky again?

Following on from a depressing adoption information evening one November night, we decided to put things off, at least for a few months. So when the doorbell rang on a chaotic January evening, we were surprised to find two social workers standing in the rain, you running around in your pants, and the dinner half-cooked. Naturally, the outcome of this 'well you'd better come in then' knock at the door was that, just three months later, our little Pickle arrived. Adopting a child because you forgot to cancel a social worker visit may seem extreme, and it was, but just like the first time – when you know, you know.

Your birthday and hospital of birth are shared with your Mama. Your baby photos resemble mine so closely it's honestly a little weird. You looked like a child's drawing of a baby, chubby with the brightest blue eyes – who could have predicted the ethereal little imp you have become, our baby bear, with the world's most delicate hands.

126

Dear Minnie

When you joined our family, any doubts we had were quickly cast aside. This time was so very different. Gone was our subservient anxiety whenever a social worker called; no, we did not listen to your foster carer who tried to convince us that you 'didn't need to nap' and that you weren't allowed to drink water because it was 'bad for you' (aged seven months). This time, it was on our terms. So, when your big sister ran at you with arms out wide in the park, excitedly shouting at her teacher, who happened to walk by, that her baby sister had arrived, I certainly wasn't going to stop to think about 'creating bubbles' and cancelling Christmas, even if your social worker was looking on angrily from the bench . . .

So now our life continues. Perfectly still again, eyes firmly on a magical future together. With one daughter who feels everything so profoundly, giving me hope that the future will be better and brighter because of the impact you'll make, and another who shows me the beauty in simply living, untouched by the doubts that others wrestle with endlessly. Your worlds are both so complicated and yet so simple, so different but so entwined, all at the same time.

What your Mama and I do know, however, is that the things we both feared in our journey into motherhood have so easily become the magic that has completed us. No matter the journey, we are perfect for each other, just the way we are.

I love you, love you and love you,

Mummy

*****

I REALLY WANTED THE PERSPECTIVE of an adoptive mum, and Faye was brilliantly candid about her experience. I have met many adoptive parents through my work and have a good friend who, at the time of writing, had become an approved adopter and had just met her little girl. Without exception, they are the kindest and most conscientious people. They go into it knowing that it will not always be an easy ride, but they are desperate to be parents, and they have so much to give.

According to government figures, 2,960 children were adopted in England in 2022–23, representing a 2 per cent decrease from the previous year. The number of children being adopted across England has been steadily declining since peaking in 2015, despite a rise in the number of children entering the care system. As of 31 December 2023, 2,410 children in England were waiting for adoption without having found a family, according to the Coram charity. This represents a 14 per cent increase from the previous year, the data showed. For the first time in recent years, the number of children in need of adoption now exceeds the number of prospective adopters. Nearly half of these children wait more than 18 months to find their permanent home.

Talking to Faye, I was reminded about the huge sacrifices some families go through to be parents and how much patience they have going into the process knowing it might take a long time.

'Looking back, so many ridiculous things happened during the adoption process,' she told me. 'There was so much I could say in my letter. These are just some snippets of our experience with adopting our kids.

'It was really nice writing it – you know what it's like day to day; life is so busy, and you don't really think about your life as a mum in this way, so it was interesting sitting down to think about what I wanted to say. I spoke to my mum and sister about the letter; we all had forgotten "the journey" and how hard it was in parts.'

Faye's two girls are five and nine, and she told us about their very different, developing personalities.

'The dynamic between them is really interesting,' she explained. 'Our older daughter is so protective of the little one, but the little one is entirely on her own agenda! They are at opposite ends of the empathy spectrum – my older one loves everyone and everything, but if the little one knew how to stick two fingers up at me, she would. That being said, she's also hilarious and so loving, we wouldn't change them for the world.'

Faye told us how hard she and her partner worked with their first little girl to do everything just right, as the social worker said, because they were so scared that something might go wrong.

'It's weird. I remember the first time we met our social worker; she was very blunt. We wondered if we should say something, but we couldn't be that person who said their social worker was borderline rude. We knew that we just had to get on with it and actually, very quickly, learnt to love her.'

We also talked about how much her children know about their history.

'As a family with two mums, there is a lot of talking.' She laughed. 'We've always been honest with the kids. We have always used the word "adoption". We've not babied them, and they have always known. Realistically, because they have two mums, there would always have to be a conversation because, obviously, we are not going to have a family in a typical way.'

Life story work is a therapeutic approach often used with adopted children to help them understand and make sense of their history and identity. Faye explained that they did a lot of life story work very early with their older daughter.

'In hindsight, I wonder if we did too much, too soon. Some of it made her quite anxious because she wasn't old enough to order and process it. So, with her little sister, we went a bit slower.'

She told me a bit about her children's history, and her older daughter's start in life was particularly hard.

'We have never once said a bad word about either of their birth families,' she said. 'That is so important, because we do not want them to build up a mystified thing. It's about being honest but not creating a fairytale alternative world. We try to keep them grounded in facts so they don't drift off. We just want to create a really emotionally safe environment for them. It's all we can do.'

We talked about the challenge of kids wanting to know more about their birth families.

'I want my children to always trust us and that we have always made decisions thinking about them above everything,' she explained. 'We tell them that our family is perfect and that to have our family, they had to have what happened to them happen. I am a big believer that there are no good people or bad people. Life happens to people, and that results in some people having to make some difficult choices and shit things happening. There is no point in apportioning blame.'

I asked whether Faye was concerned there would be a time when her girls wanted to reach out to their birth parents.

'Ultimately, it's their decision. Like everything, we can't stop it from happening, and while I sound level-headed and chill, I will find it hard. They are my babies.'

We talked about the different issues of parenthood as kids grow up, including in their teen years telling us they hate us, or for adoptive parents, the infamous 'You are not my mum.'

'I know people will see our family and wonder how we will cope with X because there are obvious differences in our family, but the truth is that crap stuff does happen to everyone,' she said. 'Our crap stuff might be different to others', and that is fine; we just have to accept that. However, in all families, it is normal to have hard, human moments.'

Faye said that even when she was much younger, being a parent was always a non-negotiable when imagining her future, while her partner felt less strongly about parenthood.

'Now, what is interesting is that she is like Mother Earth, and I love being a parent, but I love my work. I am passionate about my work [as an executive head teacher]. I love that piece of my life. So I need to do both. Once, someone asked me why I spent so many hours at school and if I shouldn't be at home with my kids. I wonder if they would've said that if I was a man? I think I am providing a strong role model for my kids, and I talk to them about the fact I am at work, but I have chosen a career that means I get chunks of time where I can be everything to my kids. During the summer, Easter and Christmas holidays, I can be mum of the year.'

Part III
Parenthood

13

'You showed me that my body can give me the greatest gift of all.'

A story of recovery

Dear Ralph,

To the boy who made me 'mum'; a name that suits me far more than Holly ever has. The love I feel for you is so powerful that I have absorbed some of it for myself. Through loving you, I cannot help but appreciate your mum, the person who gave you life; a far cry from the relationship I have had with myself previously.

I had an eight-year battle with anorexia, which, ultimately, I could describe as a failed attempt to find an ounce of self-acceptance through a path of self-hatred. From 18 to 26 years of age, I believed anorexia's lies, her protective voice that told me the life I dreamt of was a few pounds away. If only I could muster up the self-discipline to further starve myself, then I would be happy. Her scolding screams when I didn't lose enough weight and the utter shame when I caught myself in the mirror were regular parts of my day for nearly a decade. I was very good at hiding my struggles behind baggy clothes and a big smile, but eventually, I was called out by family and friends.

At the age of 23, I finally began treatment in an adult outpatient centre. My organs were in such a bad way that I had to have blood tests twice a week, and the threat of being sent to the hospital was ever-present. I didn't want to go into inpatient treatment. I was newly engaged to your dad, and we were looking to buy our first home. Yet, every time I was told, 'You must gain or maintain your weight, or you will go to the hospital next week,' I felt shame within me . . . I am too fat for hospital, then. Clearly failing at being anorexic. That was until someone asked me what I wanted out of life – not what anorexia wanted, but me. A dream of having a child was what eventually made me choose recovery.

Recovery is not a one-time choice; I had to choose it hourly. I dreamt of you constantly, and my wish for you was the only thing I could find that could compete with anorexia's fierce determination to starve me. Once my BMI was considered medically normal, we were ready to have a baby, but my body was not. It took us years. Three early miscarriages, many troubled thoughts about my body failing me and, finally, some fertility treatment before I was lucky enough to become pregnant with you. Knowing you were coming was the most elated I have ever felt. Of course, I had fears that my body would again fail us, but I hoped you would make it, and the further along we got, the more that hope turned into belief. I felt such gratitude and awe towards my body that was keeping you alive! I felt this unfamiliar pride and gratitude for and unity with my body; it wasn't failing me, and I wasn't failing it either. I was nurturing it, and it was nurturing you. I found such relief in pregnancy that I cannot begin to describe it. Food, to me, became nourishment that was keeping that heartbeat of yours going, growing your fingers and toes. Suddenly, food took on a new purpose, something to be respected, not feared.

Labour, birth and breastfeeding followed with similar amazement that my body, the one I had abused, mistreated and hated, knew what it was doing far more than I did.

I found respect for my body and its ability to do what it was designed to do. I had always felt as though my body was something to be ashamed of, but Ralph, you showed me that my body can give me the greatest gift of all – you. Staring at your tiny nose, ears, fingers and toes, and watching those familiar movements felt utterly surreal. You were here. We made it.

The lessons you have taught me have continued. You aren't even two yet, and you have taught me so much. It goes without saying that there are tough moments. Sleepless nights, big emotions (from all of us), spinning the many plates of cleaning, cooking, washing, walking the dog and making time to do all the things you're 'supposed to do': sleep when you sleep, go to baby groups, reply to messages, meet up with friends, self-care, exercise, etc. For me, there is a real challenge to that complex juggling. However, I have found that there is also a real stillness and calm in motherhood. Walking at the pace of an 18-month-old who stares at each leaf as if it contains magic is (when I let go of the idea of being anywhere on time) really 'being in the present' and actually extremely calming and very enjoyable. Play, what happened to play for the sake of it? Allowing, instead of resisting, these big emotions to be expressed has been such an education. Wow, you recover quickly if you just let out all that frustration. Who knew? A surrendering 'it takes as long as it takes' attitude is one that brings me a lot of peace these days. This is a kind of patience I have never experienced before you. Anorexia would never have had such a relaxed relationship with emotions. Anorexia protected me from feeling anything beneath the waves she created. The fear around losing anorexia was grounded in the knowledge that the waves feel so aggressive and painful, therefore what lies beneath the surface must be so much worse. But you, Ralph, with your five-minute explosive outpouring of emotions, have shown me how quickly you can just feel it and move on. How simple and yet how utterly groundbreaking.

Motherhood feels like home to me, a home that is, at times, messy, chaotic, noisy and stressful. However, at others, it's calm, peaceful, filled with love and safety and ultimately the most joy I have ever felt. I have been fortunate enough to be able to stay at home for now and not return to work just yet. I'm out of the rat race, and I'm into this slow, nurturing, maternal place with you, and I feel so alive here.

Words cannot begin to thank you enough, Ralph.

All my love,

Mum

***

Holly spoke to me about her experience of motherhood and her illness, and I felt it was such a vital viewpoint because eating disorders affect so many people, with fertility issues being one of the most common side effects. According to research, around 7 in 1,000 individuals suffer from anorexia nervosa, which is particularly prevalent in adolescent girls and young women. While anorexia and other eating disorders have traditionally been associated with teenage girls, the charity Beat reports that at least 1.25 million people in the UK are currently suffering from anorexia, avoidant/restrictive food intake disorder, binge eating disorder, bulimia, and other related conditions, affecting individuals across generations. I have met many women through my work who were suffering with eating disorders, and it is so much more complicated than it might seem.

While anorexia seems so bleak and helpless, Holly's story struck me as one that is so full of hope. Pregnancy can complicate an eating disorder as it causes weight gain and changes to women's bodies, and for many who have anorexia, I imagine this aspect is very hard. However, Holly found pregnancy to be a happy time.

'Anorexia and eating disorders are horrible, and the narrative is so negative. Yet it gave me such a different experience of motherhood, which I wouldn't have had if I hadn't had anorexia,' she said.

'I cannot describe the difference in me since knowing I was pregnant. The further along in pregnancy I got, the more I believed that it was happening. It has changed my perception of myself and the world. Who cares how small I am? I need to be looking after Ralph. That's what I need to be doing – and I need to be fuelled to do that.

'The way pregnancy, birth and breastfeeding went for me – I knew my body knew what to do and that I needed to get out of its way.'

Holly says that she'd had – unbeknownst to her at the time – disordered thinking around body image since she was a child.

'If I saw someone and I could see their ribs or bones, I would consider them really disciplined,' she said. 'That's probably been my whole life, from the age of about seven or eight.'

However, she explained that she has always been very maternal.

'I have wanted a child since I was a child. When people asked me what I wanted to be when I grew up, I would always say "a mum". That's what I wanted. I always wanted a baby.'

Holly's relationship with her body has irrevocably changed since becoming pregnant and a mother.

She told me: 'I now have pride in my body because it did something it was supposed to, and I had never felt that way. In the past, when people put on a pair of jeans, and then I put on a pair of jeans, I didn't understand why they didn't look good on me. Previously, I have always felt that my body doesn't do what other bodies do or look like other bodies do. That isn't what anorexia is about, but it is how it manifests. It's how it shows up – it beats you up for your body. The sting of that has been taken out. I look at my child, and I think that this thing I've described as a piece of shit for all my life has grown him. It's been a complete shift for me in a way that is almost impossible to put into words.

I asked Holly whether she worries about her child going through similar things to her at some stage in his life.

'For me, that is the hardest thing about being a mum – the anxiety. With him, I have done baby-led weaning because I want to make food fun. I don't want him to have a skewed relationship with food, but I am finding my feet with giving him rules. I think allowing chocolate cake for breakfast, lunch and dinner could create another skewed relationship. I don't want him to feel he has to finish food or that throwing food around is OK. It's a bit of a minefield.'

She added: 'I know that I cannot instil my mindset around food into him. I am really cautious.'

I, of course, want my child to grow up loving her body. The thought of her feeling iffy about any part of her body would break my heart.

Holly agreed: 'It would worry me more if he was a girl, as there are so many societal expectations, plus my passing down a dormant condition, potentially. Sometimes, when people talk about his "big belly", I call it his "beautiful belly", and I rub it. It's hard to know how much of this worry is because of my own experience and how much is valid.

'I heard something recently about the way you speak to yourself becoming your child's inner voice. I knew I needed to sort my shit out and that my son cannot watch me pull my stomach apart. This is such a motivation for me to sort myself out.'

We spoke about the idea of 'recovery'. Holly told me: 'There is a big debate about whether recovery from anorexia is ever possible. And I don't know where I stand on that. I think I have my life, and I am not ruled by food in the way I was. I am not all-consumed by calories. If a friend asks to meet for dinner, I will not think about whether the calories are on the menu – my first thought will be if I want to go to dinner with that person. In that sense, I feel complete recovery is possible. However, I don't ever want to stop looking for anorexic thoughts because I wonder, "If I take my eye off the ball, will she come back?" Also, now, when something challenging happens, I look out for negative self-talk.'

Holly took some time off from her career as a therapist with her son, but when we spoke, she was looking to head back to work and specialise more in eating disorders. I asked if she would have advice for other mothers who might be suffering from anorexia.

'I don't know anyone else's life, but there is a commonality in experiences for people with eating disorders, where there is this nasty voice inside your head. I can hear that. I don't know that advice is something that I could give. I think people have to find their motivation and reason for their healthy version of themselves to be stronger than the anorexic or disordered version.

'One thing that has helped me – this might not be the same for other people – is I check myself and ask myself if I would be proud of my son if he spoke the way I speak to myself. The voice I give to myself is the voice I am giving to him.'

14

'I have never seen you properly, and I will never see you properly, but I know every inch of you.'

A story of tenacity

To Isla, my beautiful baby girl,

I have never seen you properly, and I will never see you properly, but I know every inch of you. I know how your ringlets fall over your forehead, your little button nose, and what your face feels like when you smile. I never met you through a monitor screen at 12, 20, 32 or 36 weeks, but I felt every movement you made as you used my insides as an acrobatics arena. I can't find you in the crowded nursery at pick-up time, but you always find me . . . Well, you find Marco and shout my name as you hurtle into my legs, and I know exactly where you are. You're the only child at nursery whose mummy gets them there with the aid of four legs rather than four wheels. You tell everybody that Marco is special because he's a Guide Dog, and he shows your mummy where to go and makes sure she doesn't crash into people. You're not yet three, and you already know that Mummy's eyes are broken. You offer to fix them, and I explain that you can't, but it's OK because we just do things in other ways. Sometimes, I wish I could see you properly for just a minute, see what everybody else sees. But then, if I only looked at you with my eyes, maybe I would miss everything else that I know about you without even having to look.

I never knew I wanted to be a mummy until I met your daddy. Then everything changed, and I wanted you more than anything in the world. But even though I wanted you, I was so scared. I have travelled the world, I'm a barrister, and to everyone else, it seems that nothing is an obstacle for me. But the truth is everything is an obstacle that requires so much work to overcome. I was terrified that motherhood would be the same and that it would be the one time I couldn't overcome the obstacles, and I'd let you down.

Before you were born, as well as the other areas of law I worked in, I worked on cases involving children in the care system. I knew only too well that parents who have disabilities naturally fall under more scrutiny, even if, in every other way, they are exemplary members of society. Perhaps it's because people can't imagine how they would cope themselves that they automatically assume we can't or that the child will be at risk.

I went into my pregnancy knowing there might be prejudice, and I was not wrong.

At my 16-week appointment, despite having told the midwife of my job, my family support network and effectively how capable I was, I was advised that maybe I should think of hiring a nanny when you were born. Even at that stage, it was assumed I could not care for you by myself if Daddy was at work. There were murmurs of making a safeguarding referral even though there was no cause. Luckily, this did not happen, but I already felt I had to fight to prove I could be your mummy.

The rest of the pregnancy went well, although I was always guarded around professionals. I can't criticise all of them, though. Some were fantastic and never questioned if you would be looked after properly. Nonetheless, Daddy and I decided to hire an independent midwife to help after you were born to have a closer and more consistent connection and to provide us with some extra peace of mind that we were giving you the best start.

You came into this world through the sunroof. When I tell you that you lived in Mummy's tummy and then the doctor got you out, it's quite true. You were born at 9.40am on a Friday by C-section and I was glad that it was 9.40 rather than 9.39, a nice round number. Mummy is silly like that. Your entry was surprisingly quiet, given how much of a chatterbox you are now; it was just a little splutter. But that little noise was the best sound I'd ever heard.

Daddy held you first, and he pushed you back to the ward in your little fish tank. I didn't get a proper hold of you until we were back there. The first time I held you, I couldn't believe how incredibly tiny you were. You seemed so fragile, and I was terrified I would break you, but at the same time, all I wanted to do was cuddle you. I remember that first day we spent pretty much all day having skin-to-skin under a blanket, apart from when Daddy had his cuddles with you, and I often wish we could go back to that bubble when the chaos of life gets too much. We fought to latch you for a feed. We never quite got the hang of that, did we? We tried, but it just wasn't for you, despite my best efforts.

What I remember about those early days were exhaustion and paranoia. It wasn't like on TV where a choir sings, and everything drifts out of focus, and you feel an overwhelming sense of love. Don't get me wrong, I felt a fierce protectiveness towards you, and I loved you, but it wasn't the epiphany people tell you about. Mostly, I was terrified that I was getting it wrong and that other people would be watching me and judging any mistake, not as a first-time mum but as a disabled parent. It took me a long time to get over that but thanks to your daddy, his patience and the confidence he gave me, slowly I started to believe that I wasn't such a rubbish mummy.

145

And look at us now. You are a crazy whirlwind. You have boundless energy, you drive me to distraction, you are articulate and sassy and independent. But you are also so loving and funny and the centre of my world. You very succinctly reminded me the other day, when I doubted whether the bus was really coming down the road, that you have 'good eyes Mummy, the bus is coming'. Even on the days when I am exhausted from juggling work with making sure you are happy and healthy, and even on the days when we battle to leave the house on time because you won't put your shoes on, can't decide which coat you want to wear, or want to stay and watch one more cartoon, you manage to make me smile.

Daddy and I joke about what you will be in the future. He wants you to be a racing driver, and I want you to be a vet. He wants you to take karate, and I hope you will love horses like me. But, above all, I just hope you are happy and that you know how much you were wanted and how much you are loved. I hope that you never feel held back by the fact your mummy can't see you like other children's parents can, and can't do things in the same way they can. I might not immediately be able to find your favourite doll when you lose it, but believe me: I will feel every inch of the floor and pull out every cupboard until I do . . . And I promise I won't get too cross when I realise it was sitting on the sofa all along in plain sight – well, plain sight for you at least.

All my love,

Mummy

***

WHEN I ASKED HER ABOUT her sight, Kelly told me that she was born almost blind and did have some sight when she was younger.

'It's in relative terms,' she explained. 'It was never good. I could only read big lettering on a cornflakes box and never have driven a car. I was always a Braille user, had a white cane or a guide dog, and used speech software on the computer. It has got worse in the last ten years, and that's part of my condition.'

I was so interested to hear from Kelly about her experience of how professionals viewed her when she fell pregnant. I do not think it was out of malice, but maybe it's hard for someone with full sight to imagine how she would cope as a mother. When I asked her how she felt about this, she said it 'put her on edge'.

'With my job background, working with children's services [as a barrister], I know there can be unconscious bias, and I know what the results can be of that, having been at the frontline at times. I think I was probably on my guard about it anyway. You hope that it won't happen, and then it does, and it makes you very nervous, particularly as I know full well the consequences of having a red flag put on your file, even if no further action is taken.

'I was concerned that that would happen, and fortunately, it didn't, but that did put a lot of stress on me, thinking that the people I was having to deal with potentially were thinking I would not be able to manage. It was frustrating as well because I had always been very open and honest, and told them about my home life and job situation and the support I had from my family. I was constantly telling them I was capable, yet there were a couple of profession-als who disregarded that. When I told them, it was like they weren't really listening. They asked me the same questions and I was repeat-ing myself.

'I had had a couple of miscarriages before having Isla, so it was quite an anxious time anyway. People do not realise how much they could impact on your stress levels.'

Kelly explained that she felt this comes from the fact people cannot imagine how they would do it, so they assume she could not. She talked about the fact that every mother she knew, including her own, could see, so it wasn't until she met her husband, who is also blind, and reached her mid-thirties that she decided motherhood was the right path for her.

'As soon as I got to my mid-thirties, it was like my body clock told me I *needed* to have a baby and my husband wanted a family, too,' she said.

I understand now that so many mums plan when and how they are going to have kids. One of the reasons I thought seriously about becoming a mum came up when I was at the nunnery filming a TV documentary. I wrongly assumed that nuns would be square and strait-laced, but they were very sweet, and I loved their company. One of the nuns, Sister Helen, explained that one of the things she maybe regrets is having to sacrifice the idea of kids. She basically told me that I needed to crack on.

'Should I do it, Sister Helen?'

'Your career isn't going to be around forever,' she said. It was brilliant – I was having a proper life-coaching chat with Sister Helen. (This reminds me I must bring Minnie down to Whitby to meet the nuns!)

On reflection, I went into motherhood without thinking too hard about it. I know many people talk about whether they want to have a child. I think the first time Kev and I flirted with the idea, we were in this fancy hotel in north Sweden. We were having this really bougie lunch. We decided to start trying, and I assumed it would take a couple of years, but I now realise things never quite pan out how you think they might! And Sister Helen was right – my career has always been hugely important to me, and so much of my identity was wrapped up in what I did for a living, but my hand on my heart, becoming a mum has been the honour of my life (very dramatic, but very true!) and nothing else even comes close. My daughter will forever be my greatest achievement. Having her is SUCH a leveller.

Kelly talked about their first few weeks at home with Isla and the chaos that comes with adjusting to having a newborn. Her husband was able to take four weeks off thanks to paternity leave and some saved annual leave.

'We were keen to get out of hospital, so when they tried to make us stay an extra night, I just wanted to leave. In our own home, we know where everything is. My mum drove us home because I had a C-section and we didn't want to be getting the bus!

'My dad and stepmum had come round to see her because they were going away on holiday, so we arrived back home at the same time. When the door slammed shut after they left, we just looked at each other and said: "What do we do now? Get a cup of tea? Go to bed?" We stood there and wondered how we would make it through the night.

'We muddled through like any new parents do. I don't think it was any harder than for any new parent who gets thrown in the deep end. You get handed this child and told to crack on.'

When I asked her how motherhood might be different for her as a blind mum, she said she felt that she was very in tune with her daughter. Kelly relies on non-visual cues and, like other blind people, has a heightened sense of hearing and her other senses, like smell and touch.

'You use your senses differently,' she explained. 'When she was a baby, everyone used to comment on how good her bottom was because she never had any nappy rash. You can feel nappy rash under the skin – it is slightly bumpy – and the heat before it comes, so I would always tackle it with a barrier cream before it started.

'There are other little things. I would be sitting across the room and someone else would be giving her a bottle. When someone can see, I think they don't pay the same attention because they assume their eyes will do it for them, so they'll be chatting away or watching the TV, and I would say, "There's air in that teat." I could hear it and tell immediately, and tell them. I feel I am very sensitive to her emotions because I can hear in her voice how she feels or what she needs.'

As for the hard points, Kelly explained that, like any toddler, Isla wants to run everywhere. That is hard for Kelly because she can't see her.

'I was a bit naive to certain things where I thought I would be able to do it,' she said. 'I can't always take her places on my own; in certain places, I can because she will wear a wrist strap or be in the buggy. We go to a little café together and have girls' lunches. I think it's more places like the playpark and soft play, where it is not so straightforward, as toddlers don't have a good concept of risk. She's good at telling me where she is going, but at the end of the day, she is two and a half, and you can't expect her to act sensibly. If she was to have an accident and I couldn't get to her, I would worry about that. I tend to go to those sorts of places with other people. We always find ways around it so she will never miss out. I think as she gets older and understands that she can't run off, we will be able to do more things.'

Kelly uses a guide dog to help her with everyday tasks.

'Marco is my third guide dog,' she explained. 'He is absolutely part of our family. He and Isla are best friends. When he is not working, he is our family pet, and the two of them are partners in crime and thick as thieves. He follows her everywhere, loves playing with her and is extremely gentle and patient, even when she puts princess crowns and sunglasses on him!'

Marco helps Kelly navigate the outside world.

'One of his main jobs is to guide me to and from nursery, either while she walks with me holding my hand or on her wrist strap, or when I am pulling her buggy behind me in a similar fashion to a suitcase,' she said. 'He loves going to nursery at pick-up time as he knows he is going to see her. He also accompanies us to any other general kids' activities that we do.'

The juggle is real for all mums, and Kelly is no exception. She explained that she and her husband couldn't afford to not be a two-income household. She works four days a week as a barrister.

'Lawyers say that if you work in court five days, then it is really six and I didn't want to be the kind of parent who never sees their child at the weekend. I remember when I first started out, someone came into the chambers, our office, and she was really upset. Their little one had drawn a picture of their holiday, but she wasn't included in it. When she asked her why, she said: "Because me and Daddy did all these things and you were on your laptop." I never wanted to be that parent.

'I've tried to be quite strict about it,' she explained. 'She's only going to be this little for so long. She is an August baby, which means she will go to school when she is four, so I don't want to waste my time at home with her.'

Marco also helps Kelly at work.

'He guides me to and from court, regularly travels on buses and trains, and through various cities and train stations. He also has to lie quietly in court while I am engaged in hearings, although he has decided that he will often groan loudly in order to make sure we remember he is there.' She chuckled. 'Apart from that, he will assist with guiding me to the usual places: shops, family members' houses, trips into town to see friends, et cetera.'

Marco regularly accompanies the family on holidays, the most recent of which was to the seaside.

'He and Isla had a fantastic time on the beach. When he is not working, he loves a run through the fields to let off steam. As you can tell, he has fallen into a very varied and busy working lifestyle but seems to love it.'

Isla explains to all new people about their set-up – that her parents cannot see and they have a guide dog to help them.

'She is fully aware, and if I can't find something, she will grab my hand and tell me: "It's here." She is very sweet, and we have always been very honest with her.'

Kelly was very explicit about the fact that she never wanted her vision to impact her daughter so she couldn't do the things the other children did, so they would find ways to do these things.

'It really annoys me when people say she will be my carer and help me. No, she won't. I am capable, and she is a child, and I wouldn't put that extra expectation on her. She is her own person – she is smart and sassy, and I adore her.'

15

'Some days, I feel like we are battling against the tide.'

A story of strength

Dear Eddie, George and Molly,

You are quite simply the loves of my life.

Eddie, it all started with you. You changed me in a way that has altered the path of my life ever since. The moment I laid you down on that hospital bed, I knew we were going to have the best adventures together. I was scared and apprehensive. Was I good enough to be your mummy? To keep you safe? I'm still asking myself those questions nine years on!

You see, the adventure wasn't quite what I had planned. I wanted life to be perfect for you. I tried so hard to buy all the things I thought a little person needed: the White Company babygrows, the gadgets and toys. I decorated your nursery in beautiful pastels. All the things a 'good mummy' provides. I was so excited to take you to baby classes. But you were sick all over the white, the gadgets got thrown out and the toys were never really played with. I would sit in baby classes with you and wonder why other children were doing things that you just didn't seem to be interested in.

It's funny, as an expectant mother, you think that life is going to be a certain way. No one will ever prepare you for the words, 'Your child is autistic.' I thought I was heading someplace where mummies are immaculate, houses are clean and playrooms are played in. But you had other ideas. At the time, I fell apart for a little while. I wasn't sure I was strong enough. You didn't talk; you still don't, really!

I remember at your first birthday party turning to a friend and asking if she thought you were 'OK'. She obviously smiled and told me you seemed fine. Why wouldn't she? I guess. She was hardly likely to tell me she thought you were autistic. Your daddy threw you into the ball pit. Not an unusual event, as every other child was being thrown about, but something about that encounter provoked a complete meltdown. I obviously blamed it on your daddy, but even then, you were trying to tell me that the world was an over-sensory place for you to be a part of. You seemed in your own world, a far-off distant land that only you were privy to. Most of the party you spent with the string of a balloon, staring out of the window. The other children were playing alongside each other, interested in what each other was doing, eating bits from the party table. Not you. You were happy to be on the outskirts. You found loud, crowded, busy places difficult, too much to process, maybe. Or maybe you were just scared.

Every other child in the world seemed to be developing in the so-called right way, and we were on a different path. I was out of control and wasn't sure what to do with it. I was grieving the loss of a life I had planned, and that took time to make sense of. How could I be grieving when I had you? I didn't know what it meant to be autistic. I was full of fear and anxiety. The unknown can be a scary place. But at no point did

I wish you away or wish you were different. Does this make you any less perfect? No, not at all. If anything, it makes you more so. Until the sun draws to a close for me, I will fight for you and whatever it is you need in this life.

Then we were joined by you, Georgie, the boy with the biggest blue eyes and the cutest dimples I have ever seen! Another diagnosis: another battle to overcome. This time, I felt more prepared. You were the same but totally different to your brother. You would line things up and collect. In my naivety, I mistook this for 'playing'. I now know this to be a sign of autism. Fixating on certain things, organising alone, repetitive behaviours. These were all things that I 'overlooked', partly in denial, but also because you were so different to Eddie that I didn't connect the dots. They say if you meet one autistic person, then you have met one autistic person: it's so true, because everyone with autism is a unique individual. Now I know a little more about autism, it was obvious and became even more obvious as you got older. Your brother never really had an interest in any kind of toy that he couldn't chew on. More interested in the radiators or looking out of the window. It wasn't until you went to nursery that the lack of communicative language became apparent, and it was as if history was repeating itself.

You taught yourself to read at the age of two and a half! Often, people wonder how I knew this. I caught you once with a book. You didn't see me watching, but I could make out the words you were saying. It's the strangest thing when you hear someone who refuses to use language to communicate what they want or need but can read written words. You would never read on demand and still don't. If you had to interact with another person, you would shut down. That's why your iPad became your best friend. Even to this day, you prize it more than anything else; it's your gateway to the world, it's your companion, your friend that doesn't require anything from you. Never demanding, it gives up its secrets to you. Numbers, words, puzzles; it has it all in abundance.

You are eight now, and I hope that someday soon you will utter the words 'I love you' or even just 'mummy'. When you read, it's so beautiful, just like you are – my clever, smart, funny boy.

After diagnosis, and maybe even before that, life became very insular. Alone, trapped, drowning, fighting for breath, fighting for life. It is difficult to have a social life when you have children who don't conform with the 'rules'. When they are non-verbal, things become even harder. You must have complete faith in whoever is looking after them.

Some days, I feel we are battling against the tide. I liken my life to standing in a glass box, screaming at the top of my voice. People can see me, but they aren't listening to the words I am saying. 'I'm alone, I'm scared, I can't do this, it's too hard.' The challenges I have gone through every day, other people's ignorance, the failing education system, the behaviours associated with autism and the lack of support for families like ours, I have struggled. But Molly, then you came along – the light in any darkened room. You inspire me every day to keep fighting. I believe you were chosen to watch over me. To show me little segments of life which are so closed off to us as a family. We go for milkshakes and sit and watch the world go by. We walk quietly, read bedtime stories and chat about all kinds of weird and wonderful things. Things others take for granted. You give me strength, and you bring to me a balance. A glimpse at a life which I once thought I wanted. We have the best of both worlds, don't we?

When Daddy left, it was hard on Mummy. I tried not to let you see the sadness, the pure fear I felt at raising you all by myself. The sleepless nights, the cleaning poo off the wall at three in the morning because one of your brothers had smeared. I hope you still feel I did a good job. I didn't think I could do it, and then, one day, I found I was doing the impossible: raising humans on my own. The day shift and the night shift.

All three of you have given me something unique, special, surprising . . . We may not have the conventional life of others, but we have each other, we have learnt the lessons, and we stand together stronger for them. Life is about love, and we have that in abundance.

Mummy

***

WHEN I FIRST STARTED THINKING about different mums I wanted to speak with, I really wanted to shine a light on the mums and families that are not always included in the typical family narratives. I knew this must include a mother of children with complex needs and Felicity told me talking made her feel seen. There are mothers who document their lives on platforms like Facebook or Instagram, but she wonders whether people genuinely understand the reality of many mothers' situations.

She said: 'There are so many people like me. I don't particularly enjoy using social media, but the more you look, you'll see many people with similar stories. Everyone's fighting for a voice for other people to listen to. But sometimes you can tell the story, and people can listen, but they don't really hear it. They don't really have any understanding of how much mental and physical capacity it takes [to raise kids with complex needs].'

Felicity said that she has learnt to handle her situation by looking after herself over time.

'I have to look after my mind because once that's OK, some things become much easier. Healthy body, healthy mind. I just try to be positive. I don't want to be seen as a victim.'

What is life like now at home for her and her family?

'We have pretty bad days,' she said. 'I mean, the older the boys get, I want to say, the easier it gets, but some of the behaviours are more difficult to manage. For example, with sleeping, you have to have them secure at night because they go roaming around the house. They don't really talk, so it will be difficult to understand what they want and when – and that can be challenging.'

Felicity has also been on her own with her children for a long period of their lives. The kids see their father, but she is the main caregiver.

'We can't do the things that most people do. I can't take my children on holiday. I can't do it by myself. I can't do things like that. But I don't like to harp on about the fact I can't do stuff. I'm trying to focus on the things I can do. So, for example, this weekend, we spent time in the garden, doing some gardening. My eldest son likes Costa cheese-and-ham toasted sandwiches. There are times, like on the weekend, when our trip out the door has been in the car, with no shoes or socks, to the Costa Drive-Thru for a sandwich. We might go to the car wash because that's quite exciting for us, and then that is our day.'

She spoke of the mental shift she was forced to make in the early days of being a mum, when she couldn't say yes to invitations.

'When I was pregnant with Eddie, I joined the NCT group. You become that person who always has to say no. I remember them discussing organising a picnic trip to the park. I was heavily pregnant [with George], and Eddie's behaviour was challenging even when he was small. In my head, I was thinking, "I can't. I can't. I can't do it."'

Even now, Felicity described her two boys, aged eight and nine, as going in 'opposite directions' when they are out.

'I don't want to go somewhere and have the feeling that someone else has to look after my kids because, ultimately, they're not going to look after your children because they are focused on their own. I still can't go to very different places, like a soft play. If I went to a farm, my oldest would be just licking the bar of the farm gate. He is very sensory, so that is what he would be doing.'

Felicity found the right support for her two boys, who attend different specialist schools. Her first child had a playworker who supported them and found him a place at the school nursery where he still attends.

'When I walked in, I immediately thought, "He's not coming here. This isn't for him."

'I used to think so differently. There were children in wheelchairs, children with feeding tubes and children wandering around talking to themselves. That is my child. But back then, I couldn't see that, and it took my ex to say to me: "Come on, Fliss, look. That's him." I had to wrap my head around it; I had to.'

Felicity's middle child, George, is also autistic, but this presents in a different way.

'My middle guy, he's super, super bright. He taught himself to read and would say things, but he wasn't talking to you. I thought that, in mainstream school, he would learn from other kids, but it doesn't work like that. He would go in crying because he would spend all his day with a support person.

'In the end, he was given a place at the school he is at now. After a mammoth fight, with the prospect of George remaining in an unsuitable mainstream school or going back to nursery, we finally got a place in a specialist school. Fortunately for us they made a mistake and gave us another child's place. However, it worked out for both families as it wasn't our mistake and both boys received a place. Now, both my boys are in the right schools for them.'

Talking about her neurotypical daughter, Molly, Felicity says: 'She's so important to me. I'm so pleased I bit the bullet and had another child, because she brings something else to my life. We go out for coffee and a chat. She's my anchor in the world of motherhood I thought I would live in.

'She has grown up with her brothers and tells people: "Don't worry if he doesn't talk to you. It's the autism!"

'They just rub along. I think having her brothers has opened her heart up a bit more because she thinks about them. She knows not to get the Play-Doh out because Eddie will eat it, or put the Lego down in case he sticks it up his nose. She is like a little carer. You can tell they love each other in their own little ways. It's not your average family, but I'm a lucky person.'

16

'I try to remind myself these days are short.'

A story of sleep deprivation

Dear Noah,

You came into this world so wanted and loved. Your big sister and big brother were so proud when they came to visit you at the hospital.

Daddy and I were in the newborn bubble, full of love and in awe of how perfect you are. Those first few months were a blur of sleepless nights and feeding, changing and crying. It's easy to forget how brutal that newborn stage is; Mia was ten and Gabriel was six when you were born, and their newborn days were a distant memory. I remember sitting in your rocking chair, night after night, you having your milk, and playing solitaire on my phone to try and stay awake. I cherish those memories, though, as it was just you and me, our time together in the silent house while everyone else slept.

You never slept through the night; we always put it down to you being quite a small baby. You weighed 6Ib 4oz but dropped to 5Ib 14oz as you had jaundice for the first week or so. You were so cute: lots of hair and big blue eyes, olive skin just like Daddy, and tiny fingers and toes. We assumed you just needed extra milk through the night, and once you got a bit bigger, you would start to sleep better.

You got to six months and started solids. Everyone reassured us, 'His sleep will improve now he is on solids' . . . You didn't get the memo. You continued to wake, some nights just once or twice, and other nights, all night on the hour. Your cries were piercing. You have always had a loud cry. Your brother was the same. It went through me like nails on a chalkboard. Some people advised, 'Just let him self-soothe. Call out to him and tell him Mummy's here, and he will learn to fall asleep independently.'

I could never leave you crying. Every instinct in my body told me to go to you. You wanted to hold my hand to fall asleep. It made me realise how much you needed me and that I was your comfort. I knew one day you wouldn't need me anymore.

I finally gave in after countless wake-ups and brought you into our bed. We thought co-sleeping might give us an extra few hours and that you might sleep better hearing Mummy's heartbeat. I fell into bed that first night, gritty-eyed and desperate. I did not want to co-sleep. I had been through that with your older sister for two and a half years. I felt I had earned that T-shirt already and it wasn't fair I was having to resort to that again! You didn't sleep better. You wouldn't stay still and couldn't get comfortable. You kicked me in the back; you often sat up and slapped Daddy in the face or poked him in the eye; you tried to get close for a cuddle and often ended up headbutting Daddy or me, or both of us.

In the end, I had to pop a bed guard up and have you on my arm on the outside edge of the bed so that Daddy would at least be able to sleep for work. I would wake with horrible backache from lying in the same uncomfortable position all night. Even now, you are 14 months old and I still often turn to co-sleeping just so I don't have to keep getting in and out of bed. When you're exhausted physically, you very soon become mentally drained, and at times, I found it hard not to get cross with you for not sleeping and crying. That made me feel so guilty and sad, and often, we both ended up in tears in the middle of the night.

Daddy and I used to take it in turns. Daddy would take over the nights from Friday to Sunday, and I would do them from Monday to Thursday. It was hard – really hard. Daddy and I were grumpy a lot in that first year. We used to get into debates about who was more tired. This never ended well as both Daddy and I are stubborn, and we both think we are right.

I tried to go to baby classes just to get out of the house. I remember one day, the class teacher asked me if I was OK. I couldn't hold back and burst into tears. You hadn't slept for days, and I was feeling totally overwhelmed. She gave me a cuddle and told the story of her son, who also didn't sleep. She was over those days, but it helped me remember there was a light at the end of the tunnel. Other parents don't understand when you say your child doesn't sleep; unless they have a child who doesn't sleep themselves, it's hard to understand. They try to offer advice and kind words, but the fact that they have a child who sleeps through the night just makes me feel annoyed and resentful. When you are in the midst of sleep deprivation, you sometimes don't have a lot of patience.

I regularly had days where I felt like a zombie. I was living off caffeine and chocolate. That didn't help my body get back to pre-pregnancy weight, that's for sure. I felt like my brain was a swimming pool, and I couldn't concentrate on anything. I went back to work when you were 11 days old, tutoring GCSE maths in the evenings, so I had to learn to teach on very little sleep. Caffeine was definitely my saviour. During the day, I often didn't want to socialise or do anything.

By the time you got to 12 months, you still had nights when you didn't sleep. The first time you slept through was around ten months, but I didn't sleep. I was waiting for you to wake up the whole night. I remember in the morning when it got to 5am and you still hadn't woken up crying, because I was so tired, but my body hadn't allowed me to sleep. I felt so frustrated. Some nights, you were great and slept for eight hours. Some nights, you were up multiple times. There was no rhyme or reason as to why you had good and bad nights; it just seemed totally random.

I read lots of online websites on sleep. Lots of them talked about naps and overnight sleep being linked. I then became obsessed with your napping for two hours at a specific time every day. This meant we never really left the house. You did start to nap for two hours, and I felt so happy, as this gave me some time to do household chores and have some time to myself, and, at first, you did sleep well at night. But then, after about three days, you started your usual of waking up again. At that point, I just thought, 'Sod it, I need to do what I want to do for me during the day, and the night will be what it will be.'

I started back at the gym and signed us up for lots of baby classes. Your sleep continued to be hit-and-miss. I struggled to sleep even when you did sleep, as I had such high anxiety when I went to bed that you would wake up, and I couldn't switch off. It was like I kept one eye half-open on the clock, counting down the hours of sleep that I wasn't getting. That was super frustrating.

A midwife once told me sleep deprivation is used as a form of torture in military interrogations. This has always resonated with me, and I've always held on to those words and tried to remember that it's OK to cry and feel helpless. This is really, really bloody hard, and one day you won't be waking up all night; one day, you will be a young man, and instead of you waking me up all night with your crying, you will be keeping me awake all night worrying about what time you will be home, if you forgot your keys and if you are safe.

I try my best to remind myself these days are short. They seem endless at the time, but soon you will be grown, and I will look back and miss the days I had this tiny human who relied completely on me, where I was his whole world.

I love you so much, love Mummy x

***

'EVERYONE SAID WHEN YOU HAVE your third, they just slot in, and it's easy. They all lied!' Lauren laughed, after yet another sleepless night in her household and a busy morning ferrying her older children around. 'He screamed in the car, in the pushchair . . . everywhere. It felt like he never slept. It was really hard. I felt like I was going to have a nervous breakdown.'

The hardest part of early motherhood for me was the sleep deprivation. There are different things that are hard at different times, but I had totally underestimated how little sleep we would have and how it would make me feel. I've asked all my pals, 'Why didn't you tell me?' Apparently, they did!

'It's very hard to explain unless you are in it,' Lauren said. 'I think if someone told you when you were pregnant that you won't sleep properly for two years after having the baby, you might not actually believe them. You might think they might wake up but will have a feed and then go back to sleep. But then they don't. Not all the time, anyway.'

During our first year, our daughter was up every few hours, and she didn't sleep a bit longer until she was about 13 or 14 months old. It's still not consistent. Some nights, she wakes up and is awake for a few hours. She's not kicking off; she's just awake. I've got close friends who swear by sleep training; their approach is really militant, and it worked for them. For Kev and I, it was never something we wanted to do. I could never let her cry. I do think that everyone has to do what feels right for them.

Sometimes, when everyone else's babies seem to be sleeping brilliantly, it is hard not to think you are alone. While all experts agree that sleep is crucial for babies and children – and I appreciate there are countless books written on the topic! – I did stumble across one fact that cheered me up: the belief that older babies 'should' be able to sleep through the night originates from a 1950s study of 160 London-based babies, which found that 70 per cent of them started 'sleeping through the night' by three months old. However, the researchers defined 'sleeping through' as not waking their parents by crying or fussing between midnight and 5am, which is quite different from the unbroken eight-hour stretch many new parents hope for. This definition did not account for whether the babies were actually asleep during that time. Additionally, 30 per cent of the babies had not started sleeping for longer stretches by that age, and half of those who were 'sleeping through' began waking more frequently at night later in their first year.

Logically, the sensible thing to do would be to go to bed early or have a nap if they are, but then you worry that you will never do anything.

'I was up to 11.30pm watching Netflix last night,' Lauren commented. 'Noah then woke up at quarter past 12, and I seriously regretted my choices. I think you need a life and some "you" time. A bath, some snacks in front of the TV. It's what I look forward to all day.'

We agreed there is nothing worse than chatting about sleep with other parents whose children are great sleepers. On the occasions when I've met other mums who tell me their babies sleep for 12 hours straight, I can't imagine the world that they are living in.

'I've had that,' Lauren confessed. 'My eldest – my girl – was horrendous. My middle boy slept through on his own from ten weeks in his cot. I thought, "This is the life!" Then I went and had another one; he was even worse than the first one. When I was off with my middle one, the days were different when I wasn't so sleep-deprived. I'm just so grumpy now. When people say that you get more patient as you get older, that is a lie.'

Lauren talked about sharing a bed with her son to help them get as much sleep as possible.

'I don't even move,' Lauren said. 'He sleeps on my arm on the outside. All night, I am aware that he is on the edge of the bed, and I don't dare move because he is asleep. It's really rubbish.'

In many cultures co-sleeping is normal – whether it is comfortable or not. In much of southern Europe, Asia, Africa, and Central and South America, mothers and babies routinely share sleep. In many cultures, co-sleeping is the norm until children are weaned, and sometimes it continues long after. In Japan, for instance, parents or grandparents often sleep near their children until they are teenagers, likening the arrangement to a river – with the mother and father as the banks and the child as the water between them. Several studies report that most cultures around the world practise some form of co-sleeping, and very few would consider it acceptable or desirable for babies to sleep alone.

We also discussed the common argument between parents about who is the most tired. It's those low-key, pass-agg comments. In the first year, I was feeding Minnie, and when Kev understandably complained about being exhausted, I didn't believe there was a world where he was as tired as me.

'I don't think they understand what true tiredness is,' Lauren said. 'Adam – my husband – is great and will get up with him in the night, but like most mums, I do the majority of it. I am here all day, even though I am working.'

When Minnie was born, Kev had two weeks off, but then he went on tour for work for a couple of months. Of course, I understand it must've been hard missing Minnie and me, but the whole time, he got to sleep in hotels, have showers, go to the gym and hit the breakfast buffet. To me, when I was in the thick of it, that sounded amazing!

'I think there is a lot of shame around admitting you find certain parts of parenting tough,' Lauren concluded. 'I get a rage at 2am – that's the truth. It's not their fault, but it's hard.'

Lauren is right – how on earth can you be rational when you have had 50 minutes of sleep? As everyone says, everything is a phase, but sleep deprivation is next-level hard. They use it as a torture method for a reason!

17

'I hope you both have a stable life.'

A story of hope

Dear Naima and Christopher,

Growing up, I dreamt of being a mother – of having many children. Coming from a religious background where early marriage and large families were common, I dreamt of having 12 children. I can't say why that specific number, but it was a wish I held close in childhood. I grew up in Goma, in the Democratic Republic of the Congo (DRC), leaving and returning a few times before finally arriving in the United Kingdom in 2012, after living as a refugee in several countries.

Seeking asylum was a challenging and drawn-out journey. It took over two years for a decision from the Home Office, during which I couldn't work or study. Fortunately, volunteering with the Refugee Council and other charities kept me going and supported my mental health through some very low moments.

When I fell pregnant with you both, I remember the kicks were the way we communicated. If I didn't have a kick in 12 hours, I went to the hospital to get checked, just to make sure my little humans were alive in there. I spoke to you every day. As a refugee, I had no family and felt so lonely. Naima, you filled that gap from the moment I knew I was pregnant with you. You were real to me from the start, and I spoke to you all the time before you were even born. Christopher, you answered Naima's prayers for a sibling and my prayers for a bigger family. Naima kissed my bump every day.

Healthcare is what it is. As someone from Congo, where healthcare is totally absent, I am grateful. My experience with you, Naima, was wonderful when you were born in 2015. With you, Christopher, in 2021, things were more difficult; following a C-section during Covid where I wasn't allowed to have anyone on the ward with me, I had to care for you alone while still recovering in the hospital, as staff were stretched thin. I had a drip in one hand and had to use the other hand to do everything I could for you, and it was very hard. The cannula came out a few times as I sometimes needed to use both hands to look after you.

You two are my life. You are the reason I get out of bed and want to make the world a better place. You inspired me to set up an admin and accounting company that provides flexible employment for parents with young children. As a refugee, I felt that this was an opportunity to create jobs for refugees and migrants, who are often marginalised when it comes to job opportunities.

Being the sole parent has its moments. The responsibility is heavy, and I have to consult with you, Naima, to make some decisions because I'm not always sure what is right or wrong. I've mastered our morning routines, but weekends are harder. I often work late on my studies, and I wish for more help on weekends to catch up on rest. Naima, you've become my little helper – you wake up, make breakfast for yourself and Christopher, and even plan little indoor picnics to keep him occupied so I can sleep a little longer. Naima – your middle name is Angel, and this is what you are to me.

Dear Minnie

I come from a large family; I had cousins, aunties, and uncles around all the time. I wish you had that, too. I wish my family were nearby, to babysit, share stories and make weekends more fun. I grew up playing with neighbours, splashing in puddles, swimming in rivers and being free. We live in an apartment now, and though we make the best of our balcony garden, it's a different life. Christopher, you love digging in the pots, and Naima, you dream of having a dog one day, so we hope to live in a place where we can have one.

Growing up, I studied alone and managed to excel without much help, but things seem different now. Naima, you're in primary school, and I sometimes feel the pressure to achieve is a bit high for your age. You're doing well, but I want you to feel the freedom to just be a kid.

You both have opinions and don't hesitate to share them, whether I like them or not – a true hallmark of Western kids! Christopher, even at two, you knew how to speak up for yourself, telling me, 'No tell me go away!' In Africa, kids listen and obey. They don't question a grown-up, not even in a polite way.

You're growing up with so many resources: books, technology and all the opportunities I didn't have. I grew up listening to hadisi (stories) every evening and loved our vitendawili (quizzes). While those moments aren't a part of our lives here, you have so much access to knowledge and learning.

My dreams for you are simple yet endless. I hope for stability, a life where you have the freedom to move where you wish. I hope you grow into kind, emotionally intelligent individuals who make the world a better place. I pray for successful careers for you both, wherever your passions lead. I had a dream that you, Christopher, were appointed as a minister. Lots of my dreams come true. I pray that this one comes to pass! Amen! I pray that you, Naima, continue to grow confident because you are special, beautiful and talented. I hope you have deep, meaningful relationships and loving communities. Most of all, I hope you have lots of love and happiness.

Love,

Mama xxx

***

I WAS SO GRATEFUL TO hear Amina's story. I think it is so easy to forget that where we are born boils down to luck, and I think it is hard to understand the gravity of what some women and mothers have been subjected to.

I told Amina I had visited Goma and Kinshasa in the DRC much earlier in my career. It is a beautiful country.

'It was the only place I knew up until I was 19,' she said. 'The last time I went there was 2003. It is hard for me that my children cannot see where I am from.'

Amina says she speaks a lot to her children about her life growing up there. 'When my nine-year-old asks me how life was for me as a child, I always say, "very different". There are a lot of good things for kids now, but there were a lot of things that we had that were good, too. We had family and friends on our doorstep, freedom, playing . . . all those things.'

Amina expressed her gratitude for the opportunities her children have, including access to healthcare, high-quality education and a safer environment. While she acknowledged that safety could still be improved, she emphasised that it is far better than the conditions they would face in the Congo.

'I say to my daughter, "You have been born in a safe place. Never take that for granted."'

Amina noted: 'They benefit from a Western-style education, which is standard here. In Africa, this level of education would require attending a very, very expensive international school. Here, it is part of the standard curriculum and it is so important for their future prospects. The educational standards are high.'

It is also clear how much the past has affected Amina, who spoke about her mental health struggles.

'There are things that have happened that have not gone away. They leave scars, and you have to deal with them for the rest of your life.'

One of the main values and lessons she learnt growing up that she wants to instil in her children is the power of generosity and sharing. Growing up in the Congo, Amina and her family shared everything they had with those around them.

She said: 'Help those in need and don't rely solely on the government to do it. I've noticed that while people here are kind, they often expect the government to take responsibility for helping others. Change begins with you. You can make a difference while waiting for broader changes and for others to have what they need.'

Amina describes an ideal day with her kids as taking a trip to the local park and eating noodles at a noodle bar.

'We also like to go window shopping and discover things we like. If it's a warm day, we put the paddling pool out on the balcony and the children will play there. Watching them grow and develop brings me so much joy.'

Amina spoke with such pride about her children and accomplishments. 'I have two beautiful children who inspire me. I have my own admin and bookkeeping company, and I am studying accounting. We have a roof over our heads, and everything my kids want, I can give them. I look forward to the future.'

18

'My purpose was to be a constant presence.'

A story of friendship

My dearest Grace,

The first memory I hold of you is the warmth that radiated from a picture on my phone screen. You were on the brink of turning ten, a smile blossoming on your face that felt oddly familiar, as if I had dreamt of it countless times before. It was an inexplicable connection, a recognition of a kindred spirit waiting to be found or as if I already knew you.

I met your dad through a childhood friend when I was 40. The evening before seeing your picture on our second date, I sat with your dad, his voice thick with emotion as he spoke of your brilliance and strength. But there was also a profound sadness – the loss of your mother, Sarah, when you were just a tiny spark of life at six years old. A pang of sympathy echoed within me, yet your resilience and character, like a vibrant flower reaching for the sun, shone even brighter in my mind.

As we said our goodbyes on the phone that night, a simple gesture bloomed in my heart. I wanted to share a piece of my happiness with you, a tangible connection. So, I sent your dad some Liberty floral print bracelets, their colours a kaleidoscope of joy — hoping they would bring a touch of cheer to your wrist and day.

The next morning, a notification echoed quite loudly on my phone, it was so early. My heart skipped a beat as I opened the phone, and there you were — your eyes sparkling with a light that transcended the pixels on the screen. In that instant, a profound truth washed over me. I was meant to be by your side in one way or another. Not to replace the irreplaceable, but perhaps to fill a space left achingly empty after Sarah's passing.

I couldn't fathom the pain Sarah must have endured, knowing her precious time was limited, leaving her daughter without a mother's constant presence. And you, Grace, facing such immense emotional turmoil at such a young age, with words failing to express the depth of your feelings. The thought of being called 'Mum' never entered my mind. My purpose was to be a constant presence, a safe harbour where you could weather the storms of childhood and adolescence, especially after losing your guiding light.

Our connection grew slowly, nurtured by phone calls and the anticipation of seeing you for the first time. The moment our eyes met, there was an unspoken understanding between us. The day was pure happiness. We walked together along the river in Richmond. You were a little bit shy at first, but before long, we were chatting and talking about fashion and music. You were a whirlwind of energy and curiosity; your laughter made me laugh out loud. As the days turned into weeks, a routine settled in, a quiet rhythm that brought comfort to us both.

Before long, we were spending a lot of time together. The mornings were our special time. A shared smile, a sleepy hello and then a flurry of activity as you prepared for school. The afternoons were fully booked with your arrival home from school. Your bag would hit the floor, followed by a beeline to the cupboard for a much-needed chocolate snack. The kitchen floor became our stage, filled with your animated retelling of the day's triumphs and tribulations. You were an open book, sharing your joys and frustrations with an honesty that was heart-warming to me.

These afternoons were about more than just snacks and stories. They were about a connection and a space where you could be vulnerable, where laughter and tears mingled freely. We navigated the complex world of friendships, the first pangs of teenage heartbreak, the constant struggle to find your own voice. Through it all I was there to listen, to offer guidance without judgement, to celebrate your victories big and small.

One particular afternoon stands out like a beacon in my memory. The news of your soon-to-be-born brother arrived like a burst of sunshine through the window. Your joy was an explosion of pure, unadulterated happiness. The days that followed were filled with an excited countdown, your schoolwork taking a back seat to the anticipation of meeting your little brother. You couldn't wait to hold him and shower him with the love that overflowed from your kind heart. We spent hours coming up with names for him.

The age gap between you and your brother was significant, yet your bond was unbreakable from the very beginning. Watching you cradle him in your arms, a fierce protectiveness in your eyes, was a testament to the depth of your love. You weren't just a sister — you were a confidante, a protector and a friend. With him by your side, your world felt complete.

The years flew by in a kaleidoscope of school plays, science projects and whispered conversations about boys. You blossomed from an enthusiastic child into a young woman with a gentle spirit and a wisdom that belied your years.

Now, you stand on the precipice of your twenties, a young woman with a world waiting to be explored. Witnessing your transformation from a bright-eyed nine-year-old to the beautiful human being you are today has been the greatest privilege. Grace, your kindness and wisdom shine brighter than anything I have ever seen. The saying 'beautiful inside and out' feels like it was written just for you. Your strength and composure are a constant source of inspiration, a testament to the incredible wisdom you possess. I know your mum would feel this a thousand times over; just as I do. Grace, there are no words to express the immense pride I feel in the woman you have become.

All my LOVE,

C xxxx

***

I<small>T IS NOW ESTIMATED THAT</small> one in three families in the UK is a blended family or a stepfamily. Blended families are formed when a couple starts a new life together with children from one or both of their previous relationships. I feel like it is so common now, and people are less obsessed with others parenting biological kids. Loads of people have stepparents, and I felt it was really important to hear from a stepmum about her experience. Chrissy hit the nail on the head when she said: 'We all have a story to tell, but whenever I hear the word "stepmother", it feels like such a strong word. It's not necessarily associated with goodness all the time.'

I agree that while stepfamilies or blended families are very normalised, sometimes stepparents don't get a good rep, like they aren't 'proper' parents.

Chrissy told me that when she sat down to write the letter, it felt really hard. 'I feel quite blessed to have had a baby late in life – I was in my forties. I was lucky to have a son of my own – Grace's brother – but then writing to her knowing that she lost her mum when she was just a bit younger than my son is now, it brought up so many emotions. It was a way of telling me how much I love her, and even though I didn't spend every minute of the day with her, of course, I was focused on her.'

We talked about the relationship between Grace and her brother.

'They start to look after each other, and she is like the in-built babysitter.'

Chrissy talked around the fact that it never occurred to her that she would be 'mum' to Grace.

'From the minute I met her, I knew that I wasn't going to be her mum. She knew that, and I don't think that she ever wanted that either.' Chrissy became a trusted confidante instead. 'We met when she was nine and a half – it was a very good age for her because it was before she moved into those pre-teenage years. Once she started to mature, that's when I was there for her, and I could help her navigate all those many changes that happen during those years.'

Chrissy explained she was fortunate to have a job that allowed her to work from home, so she could be there at the end of every school day to talk to Grace.

'I was there for her. It was the time when I was pregnant, so I spent all my time with her. Even when my son was born, I had time for her. She called me "her BFF". That was nice, and for me, she was my BFF. She has always been wise beyond her years.'

Chrissy is from Sweden and explained that, as a Swede, it is normal to share a lot of things with your parents and friends on a very detailed level.

'I think I gave her the Swede BFF perspective on things. I think that's part of the reason she is so relaxed and comfortable in her own skin. I think she is so balanced in the way she is, and I could give her another perspective.'

As Grace has got older, their relationship has changed, but the connection remained.

'Grace going to college means we are still close but not from a distance perspective. We don't talk every day like we used to do, before school or after or in the evenings.'

Chrissy also spoke of social media – WhatsApp and Instagram – as ways of knowing what Grace is doing and connecting with each other.

'Sometimes, we send each other reels of fun things or great products that we both like. She is nearly 20 and an adult, and there are things that we can do together that we didn't when she was young. We can have a glass of white wine together, have manicures, and talk about more adult topics, like politics and TV series. I'm not talking about *Love Island*, more about thrillers and documentaries. Often, we look at the same things and can chat about them.'

She added: 'Just because we are not physically together all the time, it doesn't take away from our closeness because whenever we speak on the phone or when she comes home, we are right back where we started.'

19

'I started to imagine myself as a knight about to ride into battle.'

A story of a working mum

Dear Evie & Seb,

I want you to know about my decision to return to work.

It's not that I didn't want to spend my entire day picking raisins out of every orifice and playing, 'Where's your nose?' (Spoiler alert – it was my finger the whole time.) Sweethearts, the truth is, I thought by going back to work I'd find 'me'.

I'd checked down the back of the couch, and I wasn't there, so I must be in the office. That Nirvana with hot drinks, adult conversations and people who valued my opinion on something other than who's the best Paw Patrol *character (Rocky every time!).*

I loved watching you both grow and see your characters blossom, but I just didn't think I was enough . . . to do all the craft, painting and baking activities that would make me feel like I was the 'perfect mum'.

You both enjoyed very different things at a young age, and trying to compromise with a three- and one-year-old would have sent the best negotiators off in tears! Seb had to be let out at least once a day for a run around, and you, Evie, would take this opportune moment to get out the dreaded Play-Doh . . . 'Do you really need a multicoloured snake, darling?'

I naively believed that during the part-time hours of nine to four Monday–Thursday, I'd be Work Jo – spreadsheet wrangler extraordinaire, fixer of printer jams and Queen of the Queries. I'd be focused at work and 'Mum Jo' at home with the ability to prepare a delicious tea in the slow cooker, create a nutritional breakfast for you, and drop you off at nursery whilst sashaying into work with my smoothie and bento box healthy lunch, on time. Oh, how misguided I was!

All of the nursery settling-in sessions had been a breeze – you both loved it, and I loved it. Until my first day back in the office. Seb hadn't slept well, then we'd all overslept and were rushing out the door. Then, I was an emotional mess. You were both obviously tired, but I took everything so personally – the crying and vice-like grip on my arm. It was like there was a physical pain in my heart; I didn't want to let go, either. The superwoman at nursery managed to distract you, unclamp, remove and get me out the door. I peered back through the window and could see that you were happy, but I was alone with the next part of my day about to begin. The 10-mile stretch of unyielding motorway known as the M62 to the promised land. As I started to imagine myself as a knight about to ride into battle, I realised that maybe I needed to up my wardrobe, as navy ankle crop trousers and flat shoes doesn't really scream battle warrior . . .

I naively expected to strut back into the office, high-fiving HR, wave to the chief exec, then sit at 'my desk' and turn 'my' computer on . . . How foolish I was. I had done some 'keeping in touch' days with my manager, and the date had been settled in advance.

However, when I walked into the office, it came as a surprise to some people – namely IT. This meant I had no desk or laptop. Great! What is there to complain about? Chat to colleagues, have that hot brew you've been dreaming of – except I couldn't.

I felt really upset that I had been 'forgotten'. I didn't know what tasks I should be doing. Therefore, I felt useless, and then the guilt crept in. My mind started to race as I made my first cup of tea (of about ten in two hours). Had I done the right thing? Should I be at work? Was I any good at my job anymore? What would happen if I was late picking you up?

A cacophony of thoughts raced through my head, each one louder than the last. I felt dizzy; I needed to sit down and breathe into a paper bag. Then, my boss was there.

'Hi, yes, I'm absolutely fine. Looking forward to getting stuck in. Just one small matter of where to sit and a laptop . . .'

I'm not going to lie. There were times it felt relentless: the monotony of work, kids and home, and throw in sick bugs, sleep regression, teething and developmental leaps (WTF?!) . . . and there were times I felt lost and far from 'perfect'.

My darlings, I was looking in the past for a memory of me, a version of myself that was familiar because since becoming a mum, it was all very new, and I felt lost at times. I was worried I was getting it wrong and whether I'd ever be good enough for you.

This was a pilgrimage where I thought I'd be found in a place where my worth was measured against KPIs. Yet when I stopped, breathed and took in these moments of routine, it was you two who gave me the strength to accept that I was emerging as 'Mum'.

Love Mum

***

I FELT LIKE JO'S LETTER was so bloody relatable. When you become a mum, navigating that shift between being a mum and your working life is hard. Even now, when Jo's kids are older and at school, the juggle – as for all working mums – is ongoing. When we spoke, Jo told me that not only had she had a full day at work, but she had been roped into 'serving on the ice-lolly stall' at school after our chat.

'I've just put my mouse down; my hand is like a claw, and I'm not sure if I am coming or going.' Jo laughed.

We discussed the whole process of returning to work after having a baby. Jo is an accountant, and she was previously made redundant, which happened to coincide with when she was pregnant with her first child – her daughter, Evie.

Studies carried out by the Equality and Human Rights Commission and other organisations have shown that women are disproportionately more likely to be made redundant when pregnant, on maternity leave, or newly returned from maternity leave compared to the overall rate of redundancies among women or the workforce as a whole. New legislation came into force in 2024 that provides greater protection from redundancy for new or expectant parents.

'So, when I went back to work, it was a brand new job,' she explained. 'It was a completely different company in a completely different sector. I had to do my CV and interviews while Evie was doing her settling-in sessions at nursery. I was trying to look at my CV, but I wasn't really relating to it because, for the previous nine months, I had been a new mum. I found maternity leave really stressful because I knew I was being made redundant. I had to take Evie to the solicitors with me when she was four months old to sign the papers. Even though I knew the redundancy was coming, it still felt quite stressful when it happened. It did all eventually get sorted.'

Jo explained that during her first maternity leave, she poured all her energy into her new baby.

'At work, I am a high achiever,' she explained. 'So then, when I was on maternity leave, I thought I needed to be the "best mum". I wasn't off and staying at home with her. I was doing every baby group, getting the paints out and going to Baby Sensory.'

Once she found a new job, returning to the office was challenging because she had to prove herself all over again to a team she didn't know.

'I felt like I was having to prove my worth at the same time as I was dealing with nursery bugs and not having connections at work,' she explained. 'You make bold statements before you go off, about how you won't change, and then, of course, it does. I felt that I was not the same person as when I started the job or when I went on maternity leave.

Nothing can prepare you for having a baby, and then raising a baby that you see all day, every day, and then passing them on to someone else to look after while you return to work.

'Why can I find hundreds of books on what to do when you have kids and how to raise them, and nothing on becoming a working mum – that is a career in itself! I'm not surprised so many women end up leaving work because it is so difficult to actually get a work-life balance. No, scratch that – a kids-work-life-me balance.'

Jo explained that during her first maternity leave, her department was winding down due to all the team being made redundant, so she wasn't tempted to check in. However, when she went on maternity leave with her son Seb two years after getting her new role, she was more tempted to not be completely 'off'.

'I asked for a year off. I would've felt guilty if I hadn't taken the same time I did with Evie. I was doing projects while I was off with him on my "keeping in touch" days. I felt I needed to be there. I definitely put everyone else's needs before my own. I read on social media, "Women are supposed to raise kids like they don't work, and work like they don't have kids." The fact that this has become a normal saying like "clear as mud" and a normal view of mothers in society is crazy.'

Jo returned to work part-time because she felt like she needed to do the same for both children but found the cost of childcare extortionate.

She said: 'I worked four days a week with Evie, so when Seb came along, I felt I had to do the same. Even though I chose to work part-time, in hindsight, it wasn't financially viable because the two nursery fees were more than my mortgage, but my worth was linked to my identity then. Now it isn't in the same way.'

Recent research by an equal rights charity suggests that around a quarter of a million mothers with young children in the UK have left their jobs due to childcare pressures. The research also indicates that a significant number of women are missing out on career opportunities for the same reason. The Fawcett Society noted that more mothers are working than ever before but are facing a 'motherhood penalty' as their careers are not progressing. This follows a recent report by the UK-based National Childbirth Trust, which found that part-time childcare now averages £7,000 per child per year, with costs being even higher in London. I feel so lucky that we are in the situation that we are in and have help from family, but this is not the case for everyone. I think this country has got it so wrong.

Jo added: 'In the last 100 years women have been able to vote, can expect equal pay (yeah right!) and have careers in sectors that were men-only before. We are told we can be anything, do anything and reach for the stars at school. Yeah, great, except at some point, you might want to have kids, and as of yet, women are the only ones qualified to do this. There is a real financial quandary when you are on mat leave with your first – you don't realise the cost of nurseries until you have a baby, and then it's kind of too late!'

Jo spoke about the group of women who helped her work through the complex emotions surrounding motherhood, work and life in general.

'We go for a "rant and a run" or "walk and a wine" (if we are going past the wine shop). It's loads of women from different walks of life with different experiences, and we use this time to talk and share our stories,' she explained. We also touched on how time changes, and as

187

kids grow up and our careers evolve, our priorities shift, too. She added: 'It's only as my kids have got older that I've reassessed how I feel about work and myself.'

I remember before I had Minnie, I listened to other women talking about their return to work and I just felt that it couldn't be that hard. Surely? I wondered whether they were exaggerating. Honest to God, I now get it! Motherhood is the most demanding and most important gig for me. Now, when I go to work, it feels entirely different. Being a mum means I don't sweat the small stuff. Before, my work was always the thing I prioritised the most; now, it will always, always come second. Or even further down the list, honestly. And I am much more relaxed about things I would have previously panicked about. I have an entirely different perspective.

'I go to work for a rest, a hot drink and to sort some spreadsheets out.' Jo laughed. When I had Minnie, I went back to work after five weeks. There was a sense of urgency because one of our contributors was incredibly poorly and so, of course, there was a desire to make sure her story was looked after and finished appropriately. I wasn't ready to be apart from Minnie even for a very short period, so she came along. That was non-negotiable. Kev had gone back to work, but he was able to take the day off, and his understudy was filling in. So, Kev and Minnie were behind the camera, and my tits were leaking. That night, after having a very emotional conversation with this remarkable lady, I remember thinking, 'How on earth is this going to work? How am I going to juggle work and Minnie? I wonder if I can do this.'

But we did find our flow. When she was eight months old, I was filming in America, and we hired this trailer. Kev and Minnie stayed there while I was filming for *Sleeps Over*. Trying to juggle conversations about brothels while thinking about when Minnie next needed to be fed was new territory! It was a real learning curve. Naps were out the window, and she had no routine. Like many working mums, I was trying to figure it out, and as cheesy as it sounds, we can only give and offer our best. Looking back, I'm so glad we made that trip. When she is older, we will be able to tell Minnie about our road trip to Nevada. She will be open-minded if nothing else!

Today in the UK, women have the right to take a year of maternity leave, partners can receive up to two weeks of paid paternity leave, and shared parental leave allows eligible couples to divide their time off. Despite years of research and loads of legal adjustments, all the mothers I chat to – including my pals and through work – agree that balancing professional and caregiving roles can be tough. Jo and I talked about different approaches to work when you are a mum, whether it is working part-time or full-time, around the kids, or at home.

'When I talk to Evie about it, I explain that we all need our own time, whether through our hobbies or work,' Jo explained. 'I tell her that not only do I work for money to allow us to have different experiences, but it allows me to get my brain working in a different way to being at home. I also have my own social circle. So, in the same way that she enjoys going to school to see her friends, I also enjoy going to work for that reason.

'I think it is important to show kids that we are not perfect. I also think it is important to show my daughter that women can't do everything at the same time, but they shouldn't feel they have to. The thing I want to show my kids is a happy mum. Whether that is writing, working, exercising – whatever that is – because everyone will have their own version of happiness. For me, that's it. In the past, my identity was linked to my worth, especially when I did return to work after having both my kids, but now, after quite a few years, I am starting to realise my worth isn't linked to my work but is linked to my values.'

20

'I didn't think this kind of happiness existed.'

A story of reflection

My little boy,

Being asked to write to you and explain the profound changes you have brought to my life feels impossible. Where we stand now, in this moment in time, it felt unimaginable in the past. You're nearly two now, and never has the phrase 'time is a thief' been more appropriate.

When you arrived, life changed for the better, and that change is far-reaching. There are glimmers of joy in every day, even on the greyest, most sleep-deprived, coffee-driven, when-did-I-last-shower days. The happiness you bring touches everyone like the first warm sunset of summer. I didn't think this kind of happiness existed – not for me.

I don't remember my own childhood clearly. Home was a place of high alert and tension. My core memories feel panicked, and their soundtrack is the ringing of adrenaline in my ears. Even the good memories have an undertone of chaos. I wasn't a confident kid, or teenager. I didn't advocate for myself, excel in anything or try to stand out, until I went to college. While there, I fell pregnant and made the right decision.

I met your dad when I was 22. I met your grandad, your nanny and your huge extended family, and they welcomed me with open arms and a full glass. They were warm – an army of women thick as thieves and up for the craic. We got a dog, bought a house and got married. All the 'normal' stuff, except we didn't want kids. Then we thought we'd see what happened. Then it didn't happen. For three years. Two losses. We were on the verge of giving in, and it happened. Pregnant. There was no elation. Just a 'here we go'. Those early memories of pain, panic and instability were keeping me cold and shut off. I couldn't be heartbroken by something if I didn't allow myself to be happy.

But I loved being pregnant. It was magic. I was very fortunate to have had a very uneventful pregnancy and birth. I did a hypnobirthing course to dispel my fears, which was definitely the biggest factor in my positive experience. I loved that my body was grow-ing you, fuelled by chocolate milk and chips and dip. I stood in the shower at 18 weeks pregnant and knew you were a boy. I loved feeling (and seeing) you kick. I didn't mind having to sleep sitting up. I was OK with your foot in my ribs and the swollen ankles were hilarious. I felt so special, and I bloody loved not having to suck my belly in.

They say the love hits you when you first hold your baby. That wasn't true for me. I held you in front of me, simultaneously mesmerised by how perfect you were and scared to death that me and your dad were now solely responsible for keeping you alive and happy in today's world. It's a cliché, but being a mom really is the hardest, most important job in the world, and I was extremely unqualified. I'd first held a baby only six weeks before you were born. It took me over a week to first kiss you. I'd sit holding you, scared to show affection to this little thing that couldn't even see me, let alone judge me. Now, your face constantly smells of my spit for being kissed far too often.

Dear Minnie

Loving you is the epitome of bittersweet. As a newborn, you lay along my forearm, and I could carry you everywhere. Now, you're almost too heavy to carry and hold my hand to walk. Your babbles have turned into real words, almost sentences even. Your squishy little body is becoming lean and bony. We spent nights skin to skin, sleeping only for minutes. I was so tired, it hurt. Now you greet me each morning from your own bed with a mop of blonde bed hair and a toothy grin. I live in a constant state of grief for the baby you were yesterday, but immense pride for the little boy you are today and excitement for the adventures of the future.

The biggest change to my life since you arrived is within me. I'm trying really hard not to regret the days I spent being an emotionally void arsehole, even though I do every second! I read about matrescence, a hormonal shift women experience post-baby like a second adolescence, and it blew my mind. That, coupled with recognising the hurt, emotionally neglected and fearful child in me, lights a fire under my arse to make sure that you have a wonderful childhood and feel seen, heard, safe and incredibly loved. And that I am kind to myself, allow myself to enjoy every millisecond of your childhood and recognise what a privilege it is to be able to work on this incredibly complex project of raising a human.

Love,

Mom

***

I FEEL LIKE LAUREN'S EXPERIENCE perfectly captures the many emotions that mothers can feel on a daily basis.

'Pregnancy and motherhood are marketed either as fluffy and

wonderful, with home-cooked meals, floaty dresses and smiles all round, or a gauntlet of sleepless nights, shit, piss, vomit, saggy tits and hair loss,' she said. 'It is all those things. Simultaneously. Wonderfully boring and painfully beautiful.'

When we spoke, she was surrounded by boxes and about to move to another home near where she is based in Birmingham. Lauren – who refers to herself as 'mom' to her son Gene, like many others in the Midlands – says she does not have clear or positive memories of her childhood. She told me that she just never felt she would be a mother, let alone a good mother.

'The feelings of immense joy and pride in seeing myself soften. I am a fucking good mother. Who'd have known?! My son is incredibly happy, cheeky and playful. I cry at adverts now. Sap! The rush of love I get from pressing my face against his squishy little body is otherworldly.

'Most days, I have to shake off the impostor syndrome before brushing my teeth in the morning. Who let me have a kid?! I can't quite believe it. On the good days, I feel invincible. I went from being afraid of responsibility, hospitals and any kind of medical procedure (Botox doesn't count) to birthing a child in a pool on gas and air. I made this funny, kind and loving little human and I get to shape his childhood. And I'm good at it! Who knew?'

However, she also honestly admitted to missing her life before having kids.

'I miss my old life a lot,' she said thoughtfully. 'I miss bright, funny, rested, carefree, put-together and charismatic me. I miss having time for the gym, my husband and even the dog. I feel sad that the old me has been replaced by someone duller, frazzled, anxious, short on patience and slow to react, but I am extremely proud of who I am now. I feel valuable and powerful.'

Lauren described finding life with a newborn much easier than it was marketed to her. As someone who has suffered with her mental health in the past, she was expecting to have postnatal depression.

'Of course, it wasn't easy all the time, but touch wood, he was a great sleeper,' she explained, smiling softly. 'I watched the sun come up as I was feeding, and it was lovely. It was not nearly as bad as I thought it might be.

'Now it's harder – he is into everything. He wants to climb over everything; he doesn't want to eat what I cook him.'

I think it's the idea that everything is temporary, and I take great comfort and acceptance in the knowledge that everything is a stage. I found the first few months of Minnie's life really anxiety-inducing in a way that I hadn't anticipated. My natural default is quite relaxed. But then your baby comes along, and it's a love you don't recognise, so everything feels different.

Lauren explained she felt the same: 'I do catastrophise. I don't only need a Plan B but a Plan X, Y and Z. But I love a project, and I know this simplifies motherhood, but having a kid is the most important project you can ever have. I count my lucky stars, and I feel good.'

We also talked about the idea of social media and people's expectations of you and how you should go beyond what you think is necessary.

'It's like – you've got to do this, you have to do that, you have to prepare for your baby by doing X, Y or Z, and it goes on and on. You have to have a mould of your bump made and your boobs that you display forever in your home. Who has time for that? I work 40 hours a week! And with what money? If people want to do that, great. But I think it's not realistic for the majority, so we need to let go of any expectations in that regard.'

Lauren describes her and her husband rushing to get her son's nursery ready when she was heavily pregnant.

'We busted our guts, but I'm not sure why because we co-slept for almost a year. It was brilliant. I don't doubt that the choices that we made for ourselves and our family are the reasons why we had such a great time in the newborn phase. I know what feels right.'

When I asked Lauren how her priorities have shifted since becoming a mum, she told me: 'Priorities-wise, my son comes first. Always. It isn't even a choice I knowingly make. The shift is innate and biological. This doesn't mean that I am happy about it all the time. I feel "less than" a lot. Not as attractive or fun as I used to be. Older, wider, frumpier. A boring, snappy, emotionally void wife. That time I had to spend on myself, or just in my own headspace, has shrunk drastically. I'm not my own priority anymore, and burnout and overstimulation are very real.

'I think my values have strengthened since becoming a mother. I work in education, volunteer, and engage with my local MP and activist groups. I'm less afraid to voice concern and stand up for what is right or for those who are in need. I remember talking to a close friend at a pub years and years ago. She'd not long had a baby, and we talked about whether it was something I saw in my own future. I said no and that I felt like the world was no place for children. She said, "That's why we need more good people." That really struck me.'

Lauren also spoke about how the concept of time has shifted for her since giving birth to her son.

'Time is now more valuable than ever,' she explained. 'I get a second childhood through my son. One free of panic and worry. Sometimes, I look at him sitting on the sofa eating M&S olives and branded crisps, watching whatever his heart desires on demand, and the nineties kid in me can't catch her breath. I have the ability to create golden memories. Whether that's by holding games nights and parties for family or an afternoon in the garden with my son, drawing on the patio with chalk, eating nothing but biscuits and playing hide and seek in clean washing on the line. Sometimes memories take effort; sometimes it means letting go. Those memories and the time spent creating them are what I value most.'

Lauren credits the women in her husband's family as giving her a ready-made female network she can rely on. Her face lit up as she spoke about them.

'I don't have many friends,' she told me. 'I have one of those friends that is more of a soulmate, and I do not know how I got so lucky. I wish everyone could have a Nat. A part of me wishes I had an army of girlfriends with kids similar in age to my son, group chats and girls' nights but, where do you start? How do you make friends at nearly 40? Especially with crippling impostor syndrome, working 40 hours a week and keeping a toddler alive. But I married into a big, female-heavy, tight-knit family – the polar opposite of my own. These women look into your soul when they look into your eyes. There's no hiding and you should never turn down Irish hospitality. Will the questions they ask be slightly too personal? Probably. Will they tell you about yourself? Most likely. Do they have your best interests at heart? Absolutely. Two of my husband's cousins had babies within two months of my son being born and so we shared our maternity leave and became very close. I am beyond grateful for them, their advice and the laughs.'

She also works as an administrator for a primary school, doing the jobs of three people. She works condensed hours during term time and has the holidays off to spend time with her son, and to reduce the cost of childcare.

'Schools are very maternal, nurturing places and the people I work with are an extended family. I'm never short of support if I need to vent, ask or laugh, and my principal puts family above all else.'

Lauren added: 'I've taken myself and my son to baby and toddler groups and have always been welcomed warmly and chatted with other moms but I haven't formed any new mom friendships outside of my existing circle. We've recently moved home to a completely new area, away from our family and where we grew up, and adjusting is difficult. Maybe the change will come when my son starts nursery soon.

'I've been lucky in that I haven't had to work to build my support system. It's grown organically through extended family and work. Maintaining it can be difficult. I'd love to see my best mate more than four times a year. I NEED to see my best mate more than four times a year. I'm so bad at replying to text messages or remembering to reach out that I fear I put some of those treasured relationships at risk.'

Lauren also spoke about how she views her working life since she had her son.

'My work life has changed a lot. I used to be on top of everything and felt comfortable with my capabilities and workload. Now, I struggle with my short-term memory and overwhelm at the sheer amount of work there is to do. I can make silly mistakes and really beat myself up.

These things could be a result of becoming a mother; or maybe it's the underfunded education system I work in. I hate feeling like I don't have my shit together or am letting someone down either way. I feel like I've fallen from grace a little, but my body and brain have gone through a huge physical change, and I have to remind myself to be gentle with myself. There's a lot of talk about women being lied to when we're told we can "have it all" and I hate to say it, but I agree. Expectations are so high, and we're set up to fail.'

I finished our chat by asking her what advice she would give herself if she could go back in time.

'Lower your standards and expectations (of yourself, your baby and everyone else). Drastically. Get comfortable saying no. Instincts are real; trust them. Show your love. It's OK to give 100 per cent when you have it. It's OK to give 10 per cent when that's all you have. Everything is temporary, the good and the bad. And there should be no judgement for anyone. We all make the choices that we think work for us.'

Afterword

Queen Mins.

You are fast asleep right next to me in bed. Daddy is downstairs locking up and grabbing me a cuppa. I'm just out the bath. My most favourite part of the day is when the three of us settle in for the night when we are all at home together. It's just THE BEST.

We have had a crazy summer. We had to relocate back down to London for three months, for 'Mummy's work'. So I'm delighted to be home! You, as usual, were a great sport. I've basically dragged you everywhere with me for the past 19 months and you've adapted so bloody brilliantly. (The Nevada brothel obviously being a highlight . . .)

Nineteen months?! My baby is 19 months old! It's SUCH an overused expression but it's so on the money: the days are long but the months are short. Time is flying and you are soaring, baby. Truly. You are determined and such a little mimic. Strong and so curious. And you're crazy beautiful. You look like those cherubs that they draw on cards. We have proper conversations now and you even tell me you love me. My little chatty Pattie. My jaw dropped and my heart burst when you first said it. This afternoon, when we woke up from your nap, you told me you wanted pizza, which was less emotional, I suppose, so of course, we jumped in the car and ran to Waitrose and grabbed a pizza. I am, after all, your mum/assistant/slave.

And you know what. I said to your dad just the other night. It's all starting to feel that little bit easier. Like we've hit our groove maybe. Like we know what we are doing a little bit more. You're sleeping through now, which is a total game changer, and I'm not driving myself nuts every time you fall over or have a temperature. Together we are learning and finding our feet.

Tomorrow, we are going to the 'swings' (like we do every day) and then we will get our 'cuppa' together. And honestly, Minnie, these routines are my fave little moments now.

My best, best little pal. I adore you, baby girl. One in a billion.

I pray that when this book is out in the world (OK, 'world' may be a tad dramatic, realistically more like the UK. . .), we will have plans at least to have a pal for you to experience life with! I'd LOVE to give you a brother or sister to ride alongside. But life is mad and you never ever know what's around the corner, do you? So let's see. Let's see how much luck I've got left!

LOVE YOU FOREVER AND EVER AND EVER,

Mummy

Resources

In recognition of some of the sensitive topics discussed in this book, here is a list of resources and charities dedicated to offering support, guidance and assistance.

Infertility

Fertility Network UK

Fertility Network UK provides free and impartial support, advice, information and understanding for anyone affected by fertility issues.
https://fertilitynetworkuk.org/

The Fertility Foundation

The Fertility Foundation is the national fertility charity providing support and IVF funding to low-income couples and individuals in Great Britain and Northern Ireland.
https://fertilityfoundation.org/

Work

Maternity Action

Maternity Action is the UK's maternity rights charity dedicated to promoting, protecting and enhancing the rights of all pregnant women, new mothers and their families to employment, social security and healthcare.

https://maternityaction.org.uk/

Working Families

The UK's national charity for working parents and carers. Their mission is to remove the barriers that people with caring responsibilities face at work.

https://workingfamilies.org.uk/

Pregnant Then Screwed

Pregnant Then Screwed is a charity dedicated to ending the motherhood penalty, supporting tens of thousands of women each year, and successfully campaigning for change.

https://pregnantthenscrewed.com/

Pregnancy Complications, Miscarriage and Baby Loss

Sands

Sands works to support anyone affected by the death of a baby, to improve the care bereaved parents receive and to create a world where fewer babies die.

https://sands.org.uk/

Petals

Petals provides free-of-charge specialist counselling to support the mental health of individuals and couples who experience pregnancy and baby loss.
https://petalscharity.org/

The Worst Girl Gang Ever

A charity supporting the well-being of those experiencing baby loss and infertility.
https://theworstgirlgangever.co.uk/

Tommy's

The pregnancy and baby loss charity dedicated to finding causes and treatments to save babies' lives, as well as providing trusted pregnancy and baby loss information and support.
https://tommys.org/

TFMR Mamas

TFMR Mamas offers support groups and resources to help this community feel supported and not alone.
https://tfmrmamas.com/

Antenatal Results & Choices

ARC is the only national charity helping parents and healthcare professionals through antenatal screening and its consequences.
https://arc-uk.org/

Premature Babies

Bliss

This charity's vision is that every baby born premature or sick in the UK has the best chance of survival and quality of life.

https://bliss.org.uk/

The Smallest Things

A registered charity promoting the good health of premature babies and their families.

https://thesmallestthings.org/

Surrogacy

Surrogacy UK

Surrogacy UK was formed in 2002 by a group of experienced surrogates who believed that a successful journey for both surrogates and intended parents was one based on trust, mutual respect and, above all, friendship.

https://surrogacyuk.org/

Adoption

Adoption UK

A leading charity advocating for an equal chance for those who cannot live with their birth families, from childhood into adulthood.

https://www.adoptionuk.org/

Adoption Matters

Adoption Matters is a children's charity and one of the largest voluntary adoption agencies (VAAs) in the UK. They recruit, train and support individuals and families as adopters, and offer them ongoing support and training for as long as they need it.

https://adoptionmatters.org/

Single Parents

Gingerbread

A charity for single-parent families, fighting to create a world where all single parents and their children thrive.

https://www.gingerbread.org.uk/

SPSAS

Single Parents Support and Advice Services, also known as SPSAS, was created to help, advise and support single/lone parents.

https://singleparentssupportandadviceservices.co.uk/

Young Mums

Home Start UK

A family-support charity with expert staff and trained volunteers helping parents with young children through their most challenging times.

https://home-start.org.uk/

Down Syndrome

Down Syndrome UK
Down Syndrome UK (DSUK) is a national charity passionate about empowering parents and professionals to improve the lives of those with Down syndrome and their families in the UK.
https://downsyndromeuk.co.uk/

Down's Syndrome Association
A national organisation committed to improving quality of life for people who have Down syndrome, promoting their right to be included on a full and equal basis with others.
https://downs-syndrome.org.uk/

Visual Impairment and Blindness

RNIB
RNIB, the Royal National Institute of Blind People, is the UK's leading sight loss charity. They offer practical and emotional support to blind and partially sighted people, their families and carers.
https://rnib.org.uk/

Guide Dogs for the Blind Association
Guide Dogs is one of the UK's leading sight loss charities. Their expert staff, volunteers and life-changing guide dogs help people with sight loss live the life they choose.
https://guidedogs.org.uk/

Autism

National Autistic Society

A UK-based charity dedicated to transforming lives and changing attitudes to help create a society that works for autistic people.
https://autism.org.uk/

Mencap

Mencap is a UK-based charity dedicated to supporting people with learning disabilities and their families.
https://mencap.org.uk/

Mental Health and Addiction

Mind

Mind is a UK-based charity dedicated to providing support and advocacy for people experiencing mental health issues.
https://mind.org.uk/

Maternal Mental Health Alliance

The Maternal Mental Health Alliance (MMHA) is a UK charity and network of over 125 organisations dedicated to ensuring women and families affected by perinatal mental health problems have access to high-quality, compassionate care.
https://maternalmentalhealthalliance.org/

Action on Addiction

A UK campaign aiming to reframe perceptions of addiction, improve understanding and enable people to receive help.

https://actiononaddiction.org.uk/

Mothers Matter

A not-for-profit organisation dedicated to providing pre- and post-natal mental health support services to women, men and their families.

https://mothersmattercic.co.uk/

Change Grow Live

Change Grow Live is a nationwide charity that helps tens of thousands of people each day with various challenges, including drugs, alcohol, housing, health and well-being.

https://changegrowlive.org/

Turning Point

Turning Point is a leading social enterprise, designing and delivering health and social care services in the fields of substance use, mental health, learning disability, autism, acquired brain injury, sexual health, homelessness, healthy lifestyles, and employment.

https://turning-point.co.uk/

Trevi

Trevi is a nationally award-winning women's and children's charity based in south-west England. They provide safe and nurturing spaces for women in recovery to heal, grow and thrive.

https://trevi.org.uk/

Anorexia and Eating Disorders

Beat

Beat is the UK's eating disorder charity. Founded in 1989 as the Eating Disorders Association, their mission is to end the pain and suffering caused by eating disorders.

https://beateatingdisorders.org.uk/

First Steps

A charity for children and their families, young people, and adults affected by eating difficulties and disorders.

https://firststepsed.co.uk/

The Recovery Club

A supportive community for eating disorder recovery.

https://therecoveryclub.org/

Talk ED

Talk ED is a national, peer-led charity supporting anyone affected by any eating disorder or eating distress.

https://talk-ed.org.uk/

Refugees and Asylum

Refugee Action

Refugee Action supports refugees and people seeking asylum in the UK.
https://refugee-action.org.uk/

Refugee Council

A UK charity championing the rights of refugees and people seeking asylum.
https://refugeecouncil.org.uk/

British Red Cross

The British Red Cross helps people in crisis, whoever and wherever they are.
https://redcross.org.uk/

Cost of Living

Baby Basics

Baby Basics is a growing network of centres across the UK working to provide practical support to families in need.
https://baby-basics.org.uk/

Bloody Good Period

Bloody Good Period is a charity fighting for menstrual equity, and the rights of women and people who bleed.
https://bloodygoodperiod.com/

Acknowledgements

Every BRILLIANT WOMAN who has very kindly contributed to this book, thank you.

George, Gordon, Shammah and Albert, thank you for your continued help.